What Experts Are Saying
About Books by Lisa Morrone, PT

Diabetes

"I love this book because it takes you on a journey through diabetes and then gives you a light at the end of the tunnel, teaching how to prevent type 2 diabetes and how to reverse the prediabetic state and metabolic syndrome. Should be read by everyone interested in living a full and healthy life."

—**Mariano Castro-Magana, MD**, director, pediatric endocrinology and metabolism, Winthrop University Hospital, Mineola, New York

Overcoming Overeating

"A practical, sustainable, and results-oriented approach that will guide you to permanent mind change...*Overcoming Overeating* provides both the why and the how toward becoming the new, healthy you."

—**J. Ron Eaker, MD**, physician and author of
Fat-Proof Your Family and *A Woman's Guide to Hormone Health*

"A comprehensive remedy for weight loss. Lisa rightly views weight problems as having their origin in not just physical, but also mental, emotional, and spiritual arenas...An invaluable resource to the countless people struggling in this area of their life."

—**David Hawkins, PhD**, psychologist,
director of the Marriage Recovery Center,
and author of *When Pleasing Others Is Hurting You*

"If you have struggled with overeating, this resource will provide you with practical help. Lisa walks with you through the book... giving you a clear strategy to restore balance to your life in the area of eating. I highly recommend this work."

—**Scott Forsmith, LCSW-R**

Overcoming Headaches and Migraines

"A gift to headache sufferers and those in the health professions who are committed to helping them."

—**Howard Makofsky, PT, DHSc, OCS**
head pain expert

"A must-have for every home reference library."

—**ArmChairInterviews.com**

"A complete and understandable guide for both the practitioner and the patient...Lisa Morrone's extensive preparation, research, and years of experience are reflected in the safe and clinically proven techniques she recommends. A must-read for primary and specialty providers...and of course, anyone who suffers from headaches."

—**William Robert Spencer, MD, FAAP**
ear, nose, and throat specialist

Overcoming Back and Neck Pain

"The treatments recommended are practical, well described, and well illustrated...An invaluable resource."

—**John Labiak, MD**, orthopaedist and spinal surgeon

"Unique—it enables the nonmedical person to understand and manage their pain, but it is comprehensive enough to be an excellent resource and reference guide for physicians who take care of these problems. Well done."

—**Warwick Green, MD**, orthopedic surgeon

"A very practical approach to the key things patients really need to know. I recommend it to all sufferers from spine problems...I appreciate Lisa's treatment of every person as someone who has not only a body and mind, but a spirit as well."

—**Kent Keyser, MS, PT, OCS, COMT, ATC, FFCFMT, FAAOMPT,**
practicing and teaching physical therapist

DIABETES
Are You at Risk?
(1 in 3 Adults Are)

LISA MORRONE, PT

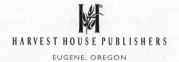

HARVEST HOUSE PUBLISHERS

EUGENE, OREGON

All Scripture quotations are taken from the Holy Bible, New International Version®, NIV®. Copyright © 1973, 1978, 1984 by Biblica, Inc.™ Used by permission of Zondervan. All rights reserved worldwide.

Cover by Dugan Design Group, Bloomington, Minnesota

Cover photo © Dugan Design Group

Graphics and back-cover photo by Peter Morrone; illustrations by Rose C. Miller

Lisa Morrone is published in association with William K. Jensen Literary Agency, 119 Bampton Court, Eugene, Oregon 97404.

DIABETES
Copyright © 2010 by Lisa Morrone, P.T.
Published by Harvest House Publishers
Eugene, Oregon 97402
www.harvesthousepublishers.com

ISBN 978-0-7369-2820-5

Printed in the United States of America

10 11 12 13 14 15 16 17 18 / BP-NI / 10 9 8 7 6 5 4 3 2 1

To my sweet children (now teenagers!),
Casey and Adam:

*What a privilege it is to be your mom!
I love you with all that I am. May the
content of this book, which we seem to have
discussed on so many occasions around
our dinner table, be a reminder to you
both to always make healthy choices when
it comes to the care and maintenance of
the glorious bodies you've been given.*

*"Love the Lord your God with all your
heart and with all your soul and with all
your mind and with all your strength!"*

Acknowledgments

Lunch on a winter's day in Manhattan with Harvest House Publishers' VP of Editorial, LaRae Weikert, is where this book idea began to take root. LaRae, you picked up on my passion for this subject, and even though I was up to my eyeballs in book contracts, you somehow managed to get me to add another! Now that this book has come to be, I am grateful, once again, for the opportunity to work with you and the rest of the Harvest House team. It truly is a message that, as you put it, *needs* to get out there!

To Peter, my husband, my friend, and my first line-editor once again: Thank you for your insightful comments and critiques of this work. My books and I are better for it.

To Mary Flanagan, my friend, physician, and medical expert: Thank you for taking the time to ensure that my research and writing was medically and scientifically sound. My readers will be blessed by your efforts.

To my Restoring Your Temple Prayer Team: Not a word in this book was written that you did not intercede for. Thank you for upholding me and my calling each week. The prayers of the saints are precious...

Lastly to Paul Gossard, my editor at Harvest House: Thank you for smoothing out this work and sharpening its message. You are invaluable to me!

CONTENTS

Foreword
by Ron Eaker, MD

Years ago Mary Poppins winsomely reminded her young charges that "a spoonful of sugar makes the medicine go down." Today it seems we have taken that advice to the extreme and made sugar the preferred ingredient in everything from sodas to soufflés.

The result? Type 2 diabetes, or "diabetes by choice," which is a leading cause of chronic morbidity and mortality in today's society. In fact, the ravages of persistently high blood sugar affect almost all aspects of people's physical and emotional well-being.

Further, University of Chicago researchers have estimated that the number of persons with diabetes will likely double over the next 25 years. And they estimate that treatment costs, in the range of $336 billion annually, will bankrupt our health system.

In *Diabetes: Are You at Risk?* Lisa Morrone effectively describes the escalating epidemic of diabetes and gives you the means to assess your own risks. She then keeps it personal and presents practical, proven tools for both prevention and treatment. Lisa knows that prevention is the holy grail of diabetes control, and the most effective deterrence begins with education. She supplies essential knowledge and then gives you motivation to translate information into action. Applying her tools and techniques will enable you to achieve balanced blood sugar, better health, and a legacy of wellness for you and your family.

Written in everyday language, *Diabetes: Are You at Risk?* guides you through the maze of information that's out there—with a medically sound approach that will help anyone adopt a healthy lifestyle by breaking the chains of fast food and bulging belts.

As a physician, I can think of no greater goal than total wellness based on a balance of mind, body, and spirit. Lisa Morrone has written a resource to help you achieve that balance. Now that's sweet!

J. Ron Eaker, MD
Physician and author of
Fat-Proof Your Family
and *A Woman's Guide to
Hormone Health*

Headed for Trouble?

Introducing a Diabetes Predictor Self-Quiz

The rapidly escalating rate at which people are becoming diabetics in the United States is of truly epidemic proportions. *One in three adults over 21 years old is either on their way toward or presently has diabetes.* Isn't that astounding?

Diabetes, for those of you who are new to this subject, comes in two forms. *Type 1 diabetes* typically begins in childhood and is thought to be the result of autoimmune, genetic, environmental, or virus-based or virus-triggered origin. There is no preventable cause or known cure for it. This isn't the type of diabetes this book is written to address.

Type 2 diabetes, on the other hand, is very often preventable. It is usually the result of years of poor lifestyle choices or neglect for which a person must "pay the piper" as they age.

In either form, diabetes is a disease process characterized by your body's inability to properly regulate the level of sugar circulating in your blood. Why is

there sugar in your blood? It's because sugar, specifically *glucose,* is your body's primary fuel source. The
human body was designed to work best when this
fuel is properly controlled by a delicately balanced
system run by an organ called the pancreas. Too
much or too little just won't do. With diabetes, there
is too much sugar left circulating in the blood, and
there is no longer an effective way of lowering it. Your
blood-sugar regulatory system—your pancreas—
is broken.

Doesn't too much sugar just make you a "sweeter"
person? No—prolonged elevated sugar levels work
to destroy your body from the inside out. The havoc
diabetes wreaks on the body is horrific. It affects
nearly every organ, from your heart and liver to
your eyes and kidneys. It can rob you of your ability
to feel things with your fingers and can cause ter-
ribly painful nerve problems, among a host of other
ailments. Its presence predicts an early and often
painful death—frequently as the result of a diabetes-
caused heart attack or stroke. And it's no longer just
a disease of old or obese people.

Because diabetes is not a single-focus disease, but
rather a whole host of health-robbing disease out-
comes, I believe it may become the United States'
greatest health threat (and medical expense) in this
next century. The Centers for Disease Control have
estimated the number of newly diagnosed diabetics

to be 198 percent greater within the next 50 years! That will nearly double today's number—from 21 million to 40 million people.

But we can do something about all this. The plain and simple fact is, *this disease can be largely avoided* if people just knew how. Why hasn't this made headlines around the globe? How come it's not on all the talk shows? I really can't answer that question, but what I do know as a physical therapist—which is echoed by my medical friends— is that, unfortunately, human nature tends toward "disease management" rather than disease prevention. We are more motivated to treat something than prevent it.

You need not wait until that fateful day when you don't feel well or a blood test comes back with unfavorable results. Your life is too precious for you to remain uneducated about the very real health threat that diabetes and prediabetes may be to you. Become the "first responder" to your own health-care issue. Time is on your side…but today more than tomorrow, and tomorrow more than next month.

In order to determine where you stand today, you'll need to make an accurate assessment of your present physical condition. Your appraisal will land you somewhere along the following five-stage continuum, which begins with health and ultimately ends with diabetes.

The Diabetes Continuum	
Healthy	You may find that you are presently free and clear of any related health issues (yeah!).
Insulin-resistant	Or you may discover that you are somewhere on the spectrum of declining health function which begins with the malady, *insulin resistance* (full discussion in chapter 3).
Metabolic syndrome	Insulin resistance then ushers in a whole host of medical problems grouped together and referred to as *metabolic syndrome* (covered in chapter 4).
Prediabetes	Of the five particular facets included in metabolic syndrome, *prediabetes* is the one which can become full-blown diabetes, given the right conditions (explained in chapter 5).
Full-blown diabetes	Most serious would be finding out that you presently have *full-blown diabetes*. But let me assure you there is hope for many who catch their diabetes problem early!

These terms may not mean much to you now, but it's been shown that even in these early stages a myriad of diseases begin and exist—diseases that used to be associated only with full-blown diabetes. That's way before a person actually becomes diabetic!

The avoidance or reversal of this destructive sequence can save your life. That's because the correlation between prediabetes and the eventual occurrence of diabetes is alarming. Scientific research has found that about *25 percent* of persons with prediabetes progress to diabetes within three to five years. Furthermore, within about ten years, *83 percent* will go on to develop diabetes unless they make some very important life changes, which we will discuss in chapters 6 through 10.[1]

Here is what to expect as we go forward. Begin by taking the Diabetes Predictor Self-Quiz at the end of this introduction. This will enable you to quickly see if you fit the profile of a person who has or could soon have diabetes. In chapter 1 you'll find a thorough accounting of all that diabetes "has to offer" (in other words, run as fast as you can in the other direction!). Next, we'll spend some time interpreting your self-quiz results in chapter 2 so you can understand what's behind the questions.

In chapter 3 you'll learn how your body *should* function to keep your blood sugar within a normal range. Armed with that understanding you'll be better able to comprehend the most common way in which your sugar-regulation system comes under attack—the problem of insulin resistance. Metabolic syndrome and prediabetes will be covered in chapters 4 and 5, and chapter 5 will include comprehensive assessment steps you need to follow to get a clear picture of where your health stands today. The second half of this book will then provide you with a detailed map that you can use to find your way back to healthier days.

Okay, enough said. Please pick up your pencil, and let's begin with a quiz...

Diabetes Predictor Self-Quiz

Place a checkmark in the box beside any
of these factors that apply to you.

Men and women:

❑ Are you carrying around excess belly fat?

❑ Do you have a close relative who was diagnosed with diabetes?

❑ Would you consider your lifestyle to be mostly sedentary?

❑ Have you been diagnosed with high blood pressure—even if it is controlled with medication?

- ❏ Have you been told you have unhealthy cholesterol levels—even if you are taking medication to improve those levels?
- ❏ Have you ever been told your blood sugar is "a little bit high"?
- ❏ Are you African-American, Native American (American Indian), Hispanic-American, Asian-American, or a Pacific Islander?
- ❏ Are you frequently thirsty?
- ❏ Do you urinate frequently (more than 8 times per day)?
- ❏ Are you over 45 years of age?

Women only:

- ❏ Have you ever had gestational diabetes?
- ❏ Have you given birth to a baby weighing more than nine pounds?
- ❏ Have you been diagnosed with polycystic ovarian syndrome?
- ❏ Does your waist, when measured just above your belly button, measure greater than 35 inches (89 centimeters)?

Men only:

- ❏ Do you have problems with erectile dysfunction?
- ❏ Does your waist, when measured just above your belly button, measure greater than 40 inches (101 centimeters)?

This is a simple test to score. If you've checked *any* box, then you have at least one, if not more, of the risk factors for diabetes. Plain and simple, you may be on your way to getting diabetes.

So what should you do first? In order to arrive at an accurate conclusion, you'll need to do a bit of investigating. I strongly encourage you to begin by reading this entire book. Take the time to absorb its message. It will empower you with everything you need to know about diabetes, prediabetes (its precursor), and metabolic syndrome / insulin resistance (diabetes' pre-precursor).

More importantly, you'll learn how you can successfully avoid the outcome that your present lifestyle and food choices may be leading you to. So let's begin!

Chapter 1

Sweet but Deadly

The Diabetes Epidemic, a National Killer

The eerie thing about diabetes and its precursor, prediabetes, is that they often exist unnoticed for many years, even decades. You live your life day by day, eating what you please, working, sitting in front of the TV or computer, and all the while a disease process is wreaking havoc at an undetected level. This "disease monster" grows bigger and more ominous every year. All he requires from you is a steady diet of refined carbohydrates and sugars.

As we discussed briefly, diabetes exists in two forms, type 1 and type 2. *Type 1 diabetes* is also known as *juvenile onset diabetes* or *insulin-dependent diabetes*. Though its cause is not fully understood, it is thought to be the result of an autoimmune disease, a genetic predisposition, an environmental factor, or an unknown virus (which is thought by some to turn the body against its own pancreas). Whichever the case, quite suddenly the pancreas is rendered unable to produce adequate levels of insulin, the blood-sugar-regulating hormone.

There is no way this form of diabetes can sneak by you for long! Most cases are diagnosed following an emergency trip to the hospital—a child is very ill, vomiting, hallucinating, or worse, unconscious. If the child receives proper medical attention in time, he or she will live.

I remember vividly the phone call I received from my girlfriend at 3 a.m. over Memorial Day weekend in 2005. Panic-stricken, she was in the emergency room with her ten-year-old daughter, who she thought was about to die! Her daughter's blood-sugar level was in the 700s (normal is 99) and she was slipping into a coma. I have never jumped into my clothes and car so fast. Thankfully, my friend's daughter lived through that frightening crisis and today is a wonderful 16-year-old.

The tough part for those such as this young woman is that throughout their lifetime, as type 1 diabetics, they'll require multiple daily injections of insulin. They'll have to test their blood throughout the day, typically when arising, before meals, and then again before bedtime—for the rest of their lives. This diligent testing allows them to accurately adjust the amount of insulin they administer and possibly the amount or type of food they eat to help regulate their blood sugar levels. Type 1 diabetics make up between 5 and 10 percent of all cases in the United States, and unfortunately, there is no known prevention or cure for their disease.

That is not so for the subject of this book, *type 2 diabetes*. Accounting for 90 to 95 percent of our nation's diabetics, it used to be referred to as *adult-onset* or *non-insulin-dependent diabetes*. Both of those labels have proven to be misnomers. Our country's rapidly rising obesity rates have now caused the onset of this disease to far predate adulthood, beginning as early as two years of age!

As for the "non-insulin-dependent" description, in the past, patients were managed solely with oral medication (no need for insulin injections). Today, often because of poor execution of diet, exercise, or self-care, many of these type 2 diabetics have found it necessary to supplement their oral medications with regular doses of insulin in order to keep their blood-sugar levels in the "safe" zone. Further, some people with type 2 diabetes have pancreases that are too far gone. They can't "go it alone" with oral medication and must therefore become *insulin-dependent*.

Later in this chapter we'll discuss a number of diabetes-related health and longevity concerns. These problems affect both type 1 and type 2 diabetics, especially those who do not keep their blood-sugar levels under tight control. However, my message in this

book is exclusively for the type 2 diabetic—the person
for whom prevention or reversal is still possible.

The Sugary-Sweet Epidemic

According to statistics from the Centers for
Disease Control (CDC), some *21 million* people
over the age of 21 have full-blown diabetes—and
one-third, or 7 million, don't even know they have
it! This is because for now they have no symptoms.
Studies suggest that the typical person with "new-
onset" type 2 diabetes has actually had the disease
for at least *four to seven years* before it was diagnosed.[1]
Take a look at the chart below, which gives abun-
dant reason for grave concern.

Diabetes Prevalence in the United States

Decade	Number of persons with *full-blown diabetes,* 21 years and older
1970s	10.5 million, or 1 in 24
1990s	13.7 million, or 1 in 18
2000s	21 million, or 1 in 12
2020s, estimated	*40 million, or 1 in 6*

Jack Challem, *Stop Prediabetes Now* (Hoboken, NJ: John Wiley &
Sons, Inc., 2007), p. 5.

Remember, every "number" is a human being
with a life to live and loved ones who care about

them. We as a nation must make a sharp U-turn when it comes to controlling the factors that can lead us straight into diabetes.

Now, why is it so important to get this book's information into your life? In a word, diabetes is a disease that, most times, *doesn't have to be!* It's *not* driven solely by genetics. You aren't helpless. (We will discuss the role that genetics *does* play in chapter 4.) Poor food choices, excessive weight gain, and a sedentary lifestyle greatly influence the onset of diabetes. Thus, you have much more control over your future than you may realize.

You want to live long and live strong. Why else would you have bought this book? So let's go forward and look this disease right in the face. Finally, let's determine that as far as it depends on us, we'll make the lifestyle and dietary changes necessary to turn us away from the diabetic destination and head toward the goal of healthy blood-sugar regulation.

What's So Scary About Diabetes?

People who have undiagnosed or poorly controlled diabetes live a sickly, highly medicated life, complete with cardiovascular disease and a high rate of lower limb amputations, vision loss, kidney and liver disease, and nerve damage—among other things. And every ailment is directly caused by the elevated sugar levels within their blood. The more carelessly a person manages their blood sugar (the more they fail to keep their sugar levels within healthy boundaries), the more numerous and rapid these disease processes become. All this damage is done by way of the bloodstream since that is where excessive sugars circulate.

Studies show that the earliest damage occurs within the large blood vessels of the body (such as plaquing and inflammation within the vessel walls), along with significant structural changes within the heart itself. These harmful effects are referred to as *macrovascular* (large-vessel) complications. Heart disease and stroke are commonly recognized examples of macrovascular disease processes that can cause sudden death.

The damage that requires much longer to show up on the radar screen as disease or disability is called *microvascular* (small-vessel) complications. These small-scale injuries, which occur within the tiny capillaries of your circulatory system, can lead to big trouble. Painful nerve damage, kidney disease, vision loss, nonhealing infections, and the death of limb tissue are some examples of this microscopic harm caused by long-term high blood sugar. Each one can eventually bring about a premature end to your life.

In addition to living with many diseases and possibly a few less body parts, diabetics are *two to four times more likely to die at any given time* than nondiabetics. Diabetes is listed as the sixth-leading cause of death in the U.S. today (up from seventh place in 2006). But consider…heart disease (for example, a heart attack) is listed way out in front of the pack at number one, and stroke comes in third. Research has revealed that physicians routinely *do not* list diabetes as the underlying cause of death on the death certificates of their diabetic patients who ultimately die of a heart attack or stroke.

For this reason alone, diabetes should hold a much higher place on the list of causes of death than it now does. I would bet, all things considered, that diabetes would come in at number three, just behind cancer. (And cancer, as we will see in chapter 4, can be "fed" by the heightened inflammation caused by metabolic syndrome, diabetes' precursor.)

Another scary thing about diabetes is how much it costs in health-care dollars. The higher the cost of individual health care, the higher health-insurance premiums rise—and that affects people who will never be diagnosed with high blood sugar! In 2007, the total annual economic cost of diabetes in the U.S. was estimated to be $174 billion. Indirect costs resulting from increased absenteeism, reduced productivity, disease-related unemployment disability, and loss of productive capacity due to early mortality totaled another $58 billion. This is an increase of 32 percent from 2002, when these statistics were last compiled.[2] The exorbitant expenses include medication, insulin supplements, increased doctor visits, medical tests, surgical procedures, and much more. If you happen to be underinsured or uninsured, diabetes can be the death of your financial health as well.

The Disease Lineage of Diabetes

Having treated patients for over two decades now, I've seen that fear of future illness can be a strong motivating factor. This kind of fear can be very healthy if it encourages you to take care of yourself and be on the lookout for the diabetes monster.

Living with any of diabetes' health issues will bring physical, emotional, and financial stress not only upon you, but also your loved ones who must take on the role of caregiver. The plain truth is that most diabetics have multiple coexisting health problems. If advanced-stage diabetes were to cause you to become a wheelchair-bound amputee, a stroke victim, blind, or a victim of kidney failure, your required care would consume the lives of your caregivers.

The truly exciting thing is, in the cases where diabetes (and prediabetes) can be avoided or reversed, many of diabetes' related disease processes can be avoided!

Cardiovascular Disease

Cardiovascular disease can be broken down into two components: *cardio* and *vascular*. *Cardio* refers to the heart tissue itself and the vessels that run directly through it. *Vascular* speaks of the vessels in the rest of your body (arteries, veins, and capillaries), and vascular disease typically refers to *macrovascular* complications—those involving the larger vessels, as mentioned earlier.

Heart disease can be multifaceted. Diabetes (and its underlying insulin resistance) can clog up the insides of your heart's vessels, much like a hair ball caught in your sink's drainpipe. This narrowing can ultimately cause both big and small heart attacks, an enlarged heart, congestive heart failure, and ultimately the failure of the heart itself. In its early stages, much of this heart disease can occur without your being aware of it. Investigators who studied a diabetic population aged 50 to 75 years found evidence that *silent* heart attacks had occurred in 22 percent of those studied.[3]

Vascular disease includes stroke, which can be caused by a sudden "lane closure" within a brain vessel. Stroke can lead to death or varying degrees of disability, all depending on the area of the brain affected as well as the extent of damage.

Another macrovascular complication, known as *peripheral artery disease* (PAD), typically affects the

circulation that supplies the legs. Known to some
as "hardening of the arteries," an associated medical
condition you may recognize is *intermittent claudi-
cation* (pain in your legs that occurs while walking
and goes away when you sit down). The many forms
of PAD can range from annoying to deadly—and
you don't get to choose which one afflicts you.

Another form of vascular disease is *high blood pressure,* which can be caused by the narrowing of arteries
outside of the heart itself. Because of the decreased
diameter of these vessels, there is an increase in the
resistance to the blood flowing through them. As
a result, your heart is forced to raise its pumping
pressure in order to circulate your blood sufficiently.
Not surprisingly, 75 percent of diabetics suffer from
high blood pressure as well (which, as you'll learn in
chapter 3, is a factor in metabolic syndrome).

The bottom line is ugly. Approximately *two-thirds*
of people with diabetes will die from heart disease or
stroke. (No, diabetes is truly not just the number-six
cause of death.) And the increased death risk does
not affect men and women equally. Among diabetics, a woman's risk of death from heart disease
or stroke is increased *three to four times* over the
nondiabetic woman, while a man's risk is "only"
increased twofold.[4]

Nerve damage

There are numerous nerve-damage problems, or *neuropathies* (pronounced "noo-ROP-uh-theez"), that accompany diabetes—from annoying tingling typically felt in the fingertips and feet, to partial or complete numbness of those same areas, to the farthest end of the spectrum, where excruciating neuropathies can cause a diabetic a lifetime of unrelieved suffering. Many years ago I treated a 17-year-old young man who was a poorly controlled type 1 diabetic. He suffered with unrelenting neuropathy in his left shoulder-blade area. Regardless of the physical therapy method I tried, nothing gave him any relief. His internal pain was unchanged by external methods.

These varying degrees of neuropathy all fall into the category of *microvascular* complications. They are caused by the toxic effect that excessive blood sugar has on the nerves' tiny endings. Overall, 60 to 70 percent of people with diagnosed diabetes have mild to moderate nerve damage.[5] And unfortunately, neuropathies tend to be permanent.

Amputations

Diabetes is the leading cause of foot and leg amputations in the U.S. In 2004, surgeons performed 71,000 nontraumatic amputations (meaning they were not done on accident victims or such).[6]

Diabetics who eventually require amputation have had years of possibly silent damage to their small blood vessels (capillaries) and nerve endings. Changes in sensation, such as numbness, lead to unrecognized sores, which often become infected due to neglect. After all, if you can't feel it, you can't tend to it. Because diabetes also brings poor healing capability, eventually these nonhealing, infected lesions lead to a completely diseased toe, foot, or even entire lower leg that must be removed.

Vision Loss

Still another microvascular complication is vision loss. *Diabetic retinopathy* is a problem with the circulation in the eyes. Starting with small capillary hemorrhages (bleeds) and followed by unwanted new blood-vessel growth, the eye's retina (the thin light-sensitive membrane that covers the back of the eye) becomes clouded. What begins as blurry vision can eventually become a complete detachment of the retina.

Diabetes is the leading cause of blindness in working-age adults in the U.S., accounting for 12,000 to 24,000 newly blind persons every year. The National Eye Institute estimates that 90 percent of cases of lost vision are preventable.[7]

Kidney Damage

Your kidneys were created with a specific task in mind—to regulate blood volume and certain compounds within your blood. They provide this service by filtering out waste products and excess fluid from your blood, regularly excreting this unwanted stuff as urine. Early-stage kidney disease can be detected by checking your blood levels of the protein albumin and the filtered waste product creatinine.

Half of all those with diabetes have some degree of kidney failure, which is microvascular in nature. The delicate blood vessels of the kidneys become compromised over time, eventually rendering the kidneys incompetent. Dialysis is required—the process of artificially filtering out contaminates from the blood. It typically requires three hospital trips per week and hours spent hooked up to a dialysis machine. Eventually, even dialysis becomes insufficient, and the kidneys fail completely. If a transplant is not performed, death is imminent.

Fatty-Liver Disease

Responsible for so many critical functions, such as filtering poison from your bloodstream, aiding in the regulation of your blood's sugar content (more about this in chapter 2), storing vitamins for later use, and producing digestive enzymes, your liver is essential. Your life depends on it. In a study presented in

Diabetes Care, an astounding 50 to 70 percent of type 2 diabetics were discovered to have fatty-liver disease, which is yet another malady resulting from microvascular complications. This disease, recognized by a disproportionate fat content within the liver, leads to *cirrhosis* (scarring) of the liver and can eventually lead to liver cancer and, ultimately, death.[8]

There's More

Persons with diabetes also have an increased occurrence of dental disease and a decrease in overall healing capacity. They suffer from a variety of skin problems and experience frequent urinary tract infections. And the foregoing pages are not a complete list by any means. When you look diabetes in the face, you realize that fear of future illness is a very, very valid motivation to make changes—changes that can vastly improve or even save your life!

You may have been wondering about the self-quiz you took earlier. If you turn the page to chapter 2, we'll now cover each question in detail and see how your answer impacts your risk of diabetes.

Chapter 2

Do You Fit the Profile?

Interpreting Your Self-Quiz

Earlier you took a self-quiz to determine whether you should be concerned about the possibility you were headed into diabetes territory. Here I'd like to explain the significance of those questions as they pertain to diabetes directly, in light of current research. The remainder of the questions—those relevant to diabetes' precursors, metabolic syndrome and prediabetes—will be addressed in chapters 4 through 6.

Men and Women:

☑ Are you carrying around excess belly fat?

Belly fat is a clear and obvious visible sign of insulin resistance, the body's inability to effectively respond to the hormone insulin. There will be more on insulin and insulin resistance in chapters 3 and 4. But for now, be aware that insulin resistance is understood to be *the* culprit behind metabolic syndrome and prediabetes—and ultimately diabetes itself.

☑ Do you have a close relative who was diagnosed with diabetes?

Between 25 and 33 percent of patients with type 2 diabetes have family members with diabetes. Having an immediate family member with the disease (a parent or sibling) increases your risk of getting the disease yourself by 40 percent.[1] Research has proven that for diabetes to be present, two things must occur. First, you must become *insulin-resistant.* Only then can your genetics "push you over the edge" into the second criterion for diabetes, which is *inadequate production of insulin.* Genetics determine whose pancreas will "buckle" under the load of excessive insulin production—which occurs when the body isn't responding to normal levels of the hormone.[2] (More on this in chapters 3 and 4.)

☑ Have you ever been told your blood sugar is "a little bit high"?

Blood-sugar levels that are "a bit high" tend to keep on climbing over the years. Higher-than-normal levels are *never* a good thing, and any fasting blood-sugar level measuring over 99 should sound the alarm for both you and your physician. Immediate lifestyle changes are necessary to reverse the situation. (See chapters 7 through 10.) So even though you do not gain the "diabetes title" until your levels reach over 126 mg/dl (milligrams per deciliter), your best chance at avoiding diabetes and steering clear of the disease factors associated with prediabetes is to heed the warning of a 100-plus reading.

☑ Are you African-American, Native American (American Indian), Hispanic-American, Asian-American, or a Pacific Islander?

Statistics gathered and compiled in the period around 2005 reveal that diabetes is not equally distributed among Americans. Your race—and possibly your subculture's eating habits—play an important role. If you belong to one of the people groups below whose population is stricken with a higher percentage of diabetes than are Caucasians— beware, and stay aware. Also, the statistics listed are for adults 20 and older. Add to these numbers the thousands of children who may, knowingly or unknowingly, already have diabetes, and I would bet these percentages would be at least a point higher per people group.

Occurrence of Diabetes by Race or People Group

People group or race	Percentage of those within group who have diabetes	Number of diabetics per 100 members of group
Native Americans	14.2%	14.2 out of every 100
African-Americans	11.8%	11.8 out of every 100
Hispanics	10.4%	10.4 out of every 100
Asian-Americans	7.5%	7.5 out of every 100
Caucasians	6.6%	6.6 out of every 100

There is a marked variation of diabetes prevalence within the Native American and Hispanic population groups. This variation depends upon a person's present area of residence or country of origin. For example, Native Americans *living in Alaska* have only a 6 percent incidence of the disease (as opposed to the 14.2 percent incidence for the entire group). On the flip side, Native Americans living in *southern Arizona* have recorded diabetes rates as high as 29.3 percent! That means nearly one in three in this group presently have diabetes. That is frightening, isn't it?

The Hispanic population (defined as having originated from Central and South America or the northern Caribbean) also contains varying rates. For example, Hispanics of Puerto Rican descent have the highest prevalence of diabetes (12.6 percent), followed by Mexican-Americans at 11.9 percent. The third most at-risk group is Cuban-Americans. At 8.2 percent, their diabetes rate ranks lower than that of the combined Hispanic population.[3]

Though exact statistics are not yet available for Pacific Islanders (Japanese-Americans and Native Hawaiians), you are considered to be at high risk because preliminary studies have established your people group has a rate of diabetes two to three times higher than Caucasians.

☑ Are you frequently thirsty?

☑ Do you urinate frequently (more than 8 times per day)?

When your blood's sugar concentrations rise, your brain is sent a message to dilute your sugary blood. It does this by triggering your thirst. In response, you drink more and more—sometimes it seems you just can't quench your thirst. The more you drink, the more quickly your bladder fills, and the more you have to run to the bathroom. If you find you are consistently having to empty your bladder more than eight to ten times a day, I believe a trip to your doctor's office may be warranted.

☑ Are you over 45 years of age?

The chance of diabetes onset increases as we age (just like your home's roof is more likely to leak the older the shingles get). By age 45, your chances of getting diabetes have risen significantly compared to when you were younger. Though age is not a major factor, it is a significant risk factor nonetheless; so much so that by the age of 60, nearly 20 percent of Americans have diabetes. That is one in every five!

Women only:

☑ Have you ever had gestational diabetes?

Studies have shown that if you have suffered with gestational diabetes during any of your pregnancies, you are not free and clear from the diabetes threat—even if your blood sugar returned to normal afterward. Gestational diabetes causes you to have a 40 to 60 percent higher risk of getting type 2 diabetes within the next five to ten years following your pregnancy, as compared to women whose pregnancies did not include the disease.[4]

In fact, a full 25 percent of women who have gestational diabetes will fall victim to type 2 diabetes within the 15 years following. Even worse, statistics show that 5 to 10 percent of women with gestational diabetes transition directly into type 2 diabetes after completion of their pregnancy.[5] This is an excellent reason to be on the alert!

☑ Have you given birth to a baby weighing more than nine pounds?

High birth weight babies put a mother at risk for diabetes, both when the child is in utero and after the birth. This factor is not fully under your control, but your best way to lessen this risk factor is to not gain more than the recommended amount of weight during your pregnancies.

Men only:

☑ Do you have problems with erectile dysfunction?

Erections are achieved and maintained when the vascular structures of the penis are filled with blood. The microvascular complications we spoke of earlier can have a significant effect on this organ because diabetes damages the vessels' walls with plaque formation and inflammation, both of which act to narrow vessel diameter. This microvascular damage, as well as increased microscopic clotting within your capillaries (a component of metabolic syndrome we'll discuss in chapter 4), can readily result in decreased blood-filling capabilities. So if your sex life is something you'd like to enjoy well into the sunset years of your life, become proactive with your health.

All of this is a lot to consider, but when you think of the consequences, your time and effort are being well spent. As we go to the next chapter, we'll look at how your body was designed to regulate your sugar levels when everything is working as it should—and what happens when things start to go awry.

Chapter 3

What Goes Up Must Come Down

How Your Body Regulates Its Sugar

As rough and rugged as some people may appear, we are quite fragile in our bodies' tolerance of swings in blood sugar. There is only a narrow window of "normal" in which your body's organs are most happy. This happy place exists when your blood contains somewhere between 70 and 99 milligrams of sugar per deciliter (mg/dl).

Really, it's a matter of pleasing "the man upstairs"—by which I mean your brain. The brain tolerates very little fluctuation in its environment. I guess you can say it's high maintenance! First of all, it hates overheating. That is why God stored it up in your cranium—away from the hot and crowded midsection of your body.

The brain's second least favorite fluctuation is in sugar. Too much can cause you to pass out. On the other hand, if there's not enough sugar—again, you'll pass out. Either way you're down for the count. If your blood-sugar level reaches an extreme on either end of the spectrum (high or low), death can result. Thus, your body was designed with a highly sensitive, highly specialized way of maintaining your blood sugar within a healthy range.

Normal blood-sugar level = 70 to 99 mg/dl

Sugar, the Fuel for Life

The food we eat each day can be divided into three basic categories: carbohydrates, proteins, and fats. *Carbohydrates* are the primary source of sugar our bodies need to survive. Carbohydrate food sources include all sugars and honey, all fruits, and all starchy foods such as bread, pasta, grains, rice, potatoes, and corn.[1] Every carbohydrate you eat will eventually—sometimes even immediately—break down during its trip through your digestive system to yield energy-providing glucose molecules for your body. Just as gasoline fuels your automobile, glucose fuels your "body-mobile."

The brain, of course, is not the only consumer of sugar (glucose) in your body—it just happens to be the one most sensitive to fluctuations. The truth is, every living cell in your body relies on sugar as its food source. Life cannot continue without it. Day and night your bloodstream transports glucose molecules as energy for everything you do—sleeping, playing basketball, anything.

Now, sugar is more than the granular white stuff in your sugar bowl.

- Table sugar (*sucrose*) is probably the best known type of dietary sugar. That's what goes in your coffee.

- *Fructose* is another common variety of dietary sugar, found primarily in fruit.

- A third type of sugar, *maltose,* is produced by brewing barley or other grains, such as in making beer. (So for those of you who enjoy beer, this could be a hidden source of sugar in your diet.)

- There is a fourth type of edible sugar, *lactose,* which is found in dairy products. (Yes, even milk has sugar in it!)

Whatever their source, all these different forms of sugar are readily transformed into glucose molecules to fuel your body's functions. So from this point on I will use the words *glucose* and *sugar* interchangeably.

Once upon a Pancreas

Blood-sugar balance begins and ends in a small, banana-sized and -shaped organ called the *pancreas* (pronounced PAN-kree-uhs), which lies deep within

your abdomen, located just behind your stomach.
The pancreas has two main functions. Ninety
percent of its mass is dedicated to the essential job
of producing digestive enzymes, which are released
into your small intestines by way of a tube called
the pancreatic duct. These enzymes are crucial for
proper food digestion.

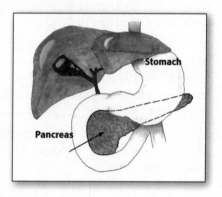

The pancreas' second function—that of regulating sugar metabolism—is what we need to
concentrate on. Throughout the pancreas there
are clusters of cells known as *islets of Langerhans*,
named for their discoverer, who saw their clustered
appearance as reminiscent of small islands, or "islets."
Although these cells account for only 5 percent of
the pancreas' mass,[2] they are almost singlehandedly
responsible for the job of blood-sugar control.

Two types of islet cells, known as *alpha cells* and *beta cells,* produce two polar-opposite hormones. *Beta cells* were created for one function: to manufacture the endocrine hormone *insulin*[3] (which lowers the amount of glucose circulating in your blood). Conversely, the *alpha cells* produce insulin's rival hormone, *glucagon,* whose sole function is to raise the amount of sugar in your blood. Together, insulin and glucagon act as a brake-and-accelerator system.

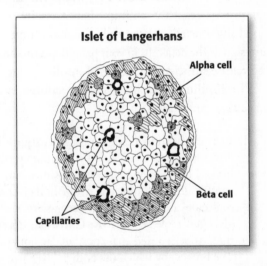

Unlike the pancreatic digestive enzymes, these two hormones do not get transported out of the pancreas via a duct. Rather, they're deposited directly into capillaries running throughout the organ, which allows them to be rapidly swept up into the bloodstream.

Life Is Good: Healthy Partnering Between the Brake and the Accelerator

After you eat, your body works to reduce all that you've eaten into three basic building blocks of life: sugar molecules, protein segments known as amino acids, and fat particles called fatty acids. The digestion process results in an immediate surge in your blood-sugar level (as it should). The sugar surge in turn signals the beta cells in your pancreas to produce and release sufficient quantities of insulin.

This insulin in your bloodstream performs two very important duties.

1. In a healthy individual, insulin acts to quickly lower any "spike" in blood sugar (apply the brakes) by changing glucose molecules into a similar substance known as *glycogen*. (If glucose molecules are the Christmas decorations, then glycogen molecules are the Christmas décor that has been boxed up for postholiday storage.) The process by which the body turns glucose into glycogen is called *glycogenesis* ("the creation of glycogen").

2. Insulin's nearly simultaneous second function is to attach itself to the body's insulin-receptor

sites. These are located primarily within your muscle, liver, and fat cells. Insulin molecules themselves have been engineered to fit the shape of their receptors, sort of like a key is tooled for a particular lock. By attaching to these receptors, insulin "unlocks" the body's "storehouse doors" so all that excess sugar, now in the form of glycogen, can be packed away for future use.

The more physical exertion a task requires, the more quickly you will burn through your available circulating glucose. When your circulating blood sugar begins to drop below normal, your brain is the first to send an urgent message to your pancreas saying, "I need more sugar!" This time it is the pancreas' alpha cells that respond to the brain's urgent call. They quickly release a dose of "accelerator" hormone, glucagon. In the bloodstream, the glucagon then acts on both the liver and the muscles, prompting them to release their stores of energy (glycogen) back into your blood as glucose—and the sugar crisis of the moment has been averted.

This reverse transformation of glycogen into glucose molecules is called *glycogenolysis* (-*lysis,* from the Greek, is a word root meaning "to release or loosen," so this term literally means "the release of glycogen"). If further glucose is needed, the liver is designed to synthesize glucose molecules from noncarbohydrate sources such as proteins and fats.

(That process is called *gluconeogenesis:* the creation—*genesis*—of glucose from a new—*neo*—source.)

Okay…take a breath and clear your mind if it has become muddled with all these details. Here are the two basic facts to take away:

1. When your blood sugar becomes too high, excess glucose is stored away for later use thanks to the intervention of the hormone insulin.

2. If, on the other hand, your blood-sugar levels drop too low, the release of the hormone glucagon enables the body's "sugar storehouses" to release some of their glycogen back into the bloodstream as glucose.

Review the flow chart below and you'll be in fine shape. One thing is for sure—life is good when these two hormones can do their jobs without interference!

When Your Brakes Fail

When the delicate balance of your pancreatic endocrine hormones is disturbed, things can get ugly. So what causes your sugar levels to rise above normal? As we've seen, when insulin is dumped into your bloodstream, the insulin receptors in your muscles, liver, and fat cells respond by accepting circulating sugar molecules for storage. We likened this to a sort of lock-and-key mechanism, where insulin is

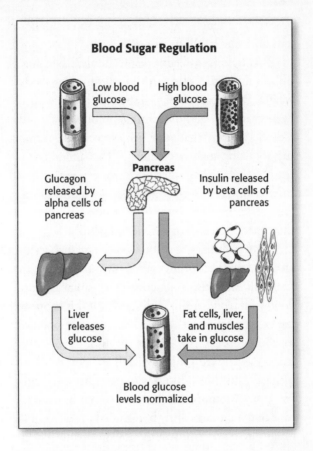

Blood Sugar Regulation

Low blood glucose | High blood glucose

Pancreas

Glucagon released by alpha cells of pancreas

Insulin released by beta cells of pancreas

Liver releases glucose

Fat cells, liver, and muscles take in glucose

Blood glucose levels normalized

the key that unlocks the receptors. This "unlocking" mechanism is ultimately responsible for regulating your sugar metabolism. In a healthy human body, insulin levels respond *in proportion* to the amount of sugar present in the bloodstream. They properly govern how much sugar will be left in circulation and how much will be stored away.

This balanced feedback mechanism becomes unbalanced most often in those with excess body weight. Being overweight—especially if you happen to be carrying a significant amount of belly fat—is a dead giveaway that your body has begun to find metabolizing sugar a challenge. This alteration in sugar metabolism comes both from ingesting too many calories at a time and also regularly eating foods that are "a piece of cake" to digest—that is, they break down into glucose too rapidly.

An overabundance of food, when digested, yields an overabundance of circulating sugar molecules. To stem this rapid rise in glucose, your pancreas must flood your bloodstream with insulin. If this happens too frequently, it eventually leads to unresponsive insulin receptors. The "cry" of the insulin molecules to store away excess sugar will fall on "deaf ears," so to speak. Just like a mom who hears her child call "Mommy, Mommy" for the hundredth time tends to tune out, these constantly bombarded insulin receptors begin to lose their sensitivity. Consistently higher circulating insulin levels, in time, give rise to the medical condition now called *insulin resistance*.

Insulin resistance is a dangerous condition. Researchers now acknowledge that it is the cause of every component of metabolic syndrome. Why is this bad? As we'll cover in the next chapter, metabolic syndrome is the road that can take you straight to diabetes territory. If insulin resistance (the forerunner of prediabetes) is not addressed with dietary changes and exercise, it will eventually become type 2 diabetes for the majority of people. You'll move from insulin-resistant to "insulin-defiant."

And what's the issue with high blood sugar? The higher your levels get, the thicker your blood becomes. Thicker blood moves through your vessels more slowly and takes much greater effort by your heart to pump. Did you know that if your blood sugar level rises too high, your blood takes on the consistency of the heavy syrup in a can of peaches? Try pumping *that* through your capillaries! Syrupy blood, to any degree, puts you at increased risk for heart attack and stroke—not to mention all the other bad-boy diseases we talked about in chapter 1.

I've provided flowcharts below to summarize and contrast healthy and unhealthy sugar regulation. Take your time as you read through them. Your good understanding will form a strong foundation for the health turnaround you can experience as you put this book's final chapters into action. After all, it may be that you're causing your own brakes to fail.

In the next two chapters, as you examine in detail the downslope route from healthy, "life is good" sugar regulation to out-of-control glucose levels, you'll start to grasp how to protect yourself from such destruction and even reverse much of the damage that may have already occurred.

**Normal Blood-Sugar Regulation
in the Healthy Person**

Blood sugar drops, indicating a need for refueling

Brain sends the "I need food"
message, and food is eaten

Digestive system breaks down food into
glucose (basic sugar molecules)

Blood sugar begins to rise

Pancreas secretes insulin to prevent the
body's sugar level from getting too high

Excess circulating blood sugar is stored
away in muscle, liver, and fat cells

Two to three hours later, blood sugar
levels off at "normal"—99 or below

Attempted Blood-Sugar Regulation in the Insulin-Resistant Person

Low, normal, or possibly even excessive circulating blood sugar

⬇

Food eaten

⬇

Digestive system breaks down food into glucose (basic sugar molecules)

⬇

Blood sugar begins to spike

⬇

Insulin is released in excess (from an over-worked pancreas) in an attempt to stimulate the dulled insulin receptors to respond

⬇

Insulin receptors in the fat, liver, and muscle cells moderately and sluggishly comply with the request to store away glucose

⬇

Blood sugar lowers very slowly, remaining high for far too long

⬇

Blood-sugar levels may eventually return to normal, but in more progressed cases, they stay elevated

Chapter 4

The Road to Diabetes

Understanding Metabolic Syndrome

Now that you have a grasp on how your body's function becomes unfavorably altered when excessive insulin production leads to insulin resistance, let's follow the disease process to its next phase. As mentioned earlier, there exists a precursory stage on the way to diabetes called *metabolic syndrome (MBS)*. This syndrome—something to fear in itself—can lead straight into diabetes territory.

According to the National Heart, Lung, and Blood Institute, a full 85 percent of those with type 2 diabetes have MBS as well. Study findings such as these clearly support the fact that most type 2 diabetics have found their way to diabetes by way of metabolic syndrome. This chapter will enable you to recognize the signs of metabolic syndrome, and then in the next two chapters you'll learn how to determine whether you're already there.

What does *metabolic syndrome* actually mean? The first word, *metabolic,* refers to the process of metabolism, which essentially is the way your body turns food sources (ultimately glucose molecules) into energy. The next term, *syndrome,* is used in medicine when describing a group of related but separate abnormalities. For example, in my professional field of physical therapy, *postural syndrome* refers to pain caused by abnormal, misaligned posture. It can have many components, such as a forward-held head position, rounded shoulders, flattened lower back, and so on. Similarly, metabolic syndrome can be described as a group of separate yet related abnormalities, each of which have been brought about by the body's inability (because of insulin resistance) to properly process sugar into energy.

The Five Distinct Markers of Metabolic Syndrome

In my earlier book *Overcoming Overeating,* I explained the five features of metabolic syndrome in a chapter entitled "The High Cost of Overweight."[1] Below is an expanded discussion of this crucial topic. If you have read my previous book, please don't skip this section—it will give you a more thorough understanding of the subject.

MBS Marker #1—Altered / Elevated Levels of Circulating Fats

Fats that circulate within your bloodstream are collectively called *lipids.* In and of themselves, these circulating fats are neither good nor bad. It is when they overstep their boundaries that trouble begins. We've all heard of *HDLs* and *LDLs*. The job of HDLs—high-density lipoproteins ("good" cholesterol)—is to carry LDLs—low-density lipoproteins ("bad" cholesterol) away from the walls of the arteries and dump them back into the bloodstream. This action prevents the buildup of cholesterol within the artery walls.

HDLs are now known to exist in various sizes. The larger the particle size, the better cleanup job they do. When HDL levels drop below the level of 40 mg/dl in men and below 50 mg/dl in women, you lose that anticlogging, Drano benefit. This condition grants you the metabolic syndrome "Seal of Disapproval" in this category.

Other things to know about fats in your bloodstream. Other unwanted alterations in circulating fats are not MBS markers per se, but they certainly show increased risk of heart disease and stroke. One of these negatives is elevated levels of the harmful lipids—LDLs and *triglycerides*. Think of these fat particles as rough rocks circulating through your vessels at high speed, banging into the walls, creating nicks and cuts.

Many times, the particles hit vessel walls with enough force that they actually become embedded in the lining. Your body's natural response to these wounds is inflammation or swelling. But it gets worse. More LDL and triglyceride particles adhere to these swollen areas, further obstructing blood flow! "Ambulance cells" (macrophages, one kind of white blood cell) rush to the site in an attempt to repair this damage, and ultimately they lay down more smooth muscle cells as a bandage of sorts. Both the initial damage and the subsequent repair narrow your blood vessels, which eventually leads to higher blood pressure and possible blockage.

Even more important than the overall numbers of circulating LDL molecules are their size. The latest information is that the smaller the LDL particle size, the more harmful it is. Smaller particles more readily embed themselves in your vessel walls. Many cardiologists now analyze both your amount of LDLs and also the actual type or size of the particles. This has proven to be a better prediction of your overall cardiovascular risk.

Finally, with documented cardiovascular disease, LDL levels are typically frowned upon when they rise above 70 mg/dl, though some variation exists between male and female patients. Triglyceride levels are considered to be unsafe when elevated beyond 150 mg/dl. LDL, triglyceride, and HDL levels can all be determined with a simple blood test (see chapter 5).

MBS Marker #2—High Blood Pressure

Your blood pressure measurement has two elements. The first, or "top," number is the *systolic* measurement—the highest pressure, which occurs when your heart contracts and pushes blood into your arteries. The second, or "bottom," number is the *diastolic* measurement, which is the remaining pressure within your arteries when your heart relaxes and fills back up with blood. Normal blood pressure should be at or less than 120/80 mmHg (millimeters of mercury, referring to older-style measuring equipment).

Clinically speaking, high blood pressure is anything over 140/90 mmHg. Medical professionals call this hypertension (HTN). If your blood pressure lies between normal and high (121 to 139 / 81 to 89 mm/Hg) then you fall into the category of *prehypertension*—an area where extreme caution and lifestyle changes should be pursued.

All that said, blood pressure registering at *130/85 mm/Hg or greater* warrants the diagnosis of MBS, according to the National Heart, Lung, and Blood Institute.

Elevated blood pressure increases the turbulence (or speed and agitation) of your blood flow. This "whitewater rapids" flow causes vessel-wall damage by speeding up the abrasive circulating substances (the lipids discussed above, as well as your own blood cells). As mentioned in chapter 1, high blood pressure takes a toll on your heart and other organs over time, increasing your risk of stroke or heart attack, as well as kidney damage or failure.

MBS Marker #3—High Blood-Sugar Levels

Healthy blood-sugar levels range between 70 and 99 mg/dl, which reflects normal fluctuation in circulating glucose. Levels are most accurately measured after a ten-to-twelve-hour period of fasting (say, first thing in the morning) or two to three hours following your last meal or snack. *Prediabetes* is diagnosed when your level is detected to be between 100 and 125 mg/dl.

In my experience, some patients and their doctors don't take this early warning seriously enough. Not so with my friend, Karen, and her physician. The very day she was confronted with the diagnosis of elevated blood sugar, her doctor suggested medication, and Karen started out on the road to recovery (which required dedication to weight loss, a healthy diet, and regular exercise). It took her only a few months to exchange her rise in blood sugar for a drop. In fact, her sugar dropped so significantly that her doctor said she could stop taking the medication!

Medications are helpful in managing blood-sugar problems, but it is always best, when possible, to not resort to "management" but to rid yourself of your problem naturally. (See chapters 7 through 10.) All medications come with baggage—side effects such as liver damage, and so on. Why go there if you can successfully "go it alone"?*

Diagnostic Fasting Blood-Sugar Levels

Normal	Prediabetes	Diabetes
Less than 99 mg/dl	100 to 125 mg/dl	More than 126 mg/dl

Keep in mind that increased levels of blood sugar first occur when you're developing insulin resistance. The problem with waiting to do something is that insulin resistance takes its toll in many ways *before* you get diabetes—and even if you never progress into full-blown diabetes. But time is on your side. Just like early cancer detection is strongly emphasized, I hope early rise in blood-sugar levels will follow suit. It can be nearly as deadly!

MBS Marker #4—A State of Increased Risk of Clotting

Also known as a *pro-thrombotic* state, a state of increased risk for blood clots (and therefore vessel

---

* I am not suggesting that you ignore doctor's orders to medicate. Follow Karen's example and allow the medication to be your protection *while* you are enacting change. Also, sometimes diabetes is too far advanced to normalize blood sugar with lifestyle changes alone. In these cases, medicine along with lifestyle changes is your best approach (see chapter 10).

clogging) is harmful for the simple reason that a "logjam" inside a vessel is a bad thing. If it occurs in a limb, you can lose the limb; if it occurs in your heart, you'll experience an oxygen and fuel shortage in your heart resulting in angina (chest pain), or worse, a heart attack. And if a vessel within your brain becomes clogged, you suffer a stroke.

Many years ago I treated a patient who was an overweight smoker. Although she was in physical therapy for a neck issue, she complained that her left hand always felt cold. Whenever I felt it, I never perceived a temperature difference—until one day. It was so very cold that I immediately took her wrist pulse—that is, I *attempted* to take her pulse. It was not there! I sent her directly to her doctor, who scheduled emergency surgery after detecting a clogged artery in her left lower neck area. She returned to physical therapy the next week with a surgical bandage across her neck and a smile across her face. The timely diagnosis and surgery had saved her arm! Close call…too close for both of us. (By the way, smoking has been found to increase insulin resistance.)

MBS Marker #5—A State of Heightened Inflammation

A *pro-inflammatory state* is, loosely, a chemically related situation that "irritates" many of the cells of your body. When the lining of your blood vessels is in this inflamed or aggravated state, it has an over-reactive response to the abrasion injuries mentioned earlier. (When you're in a bad mood, don't you tend to overreact to small insults as well?) The resulting excessive inflammation going on within your vessel walls adds insult to injury as far as vascular and heart disease is concerned.

Numerous inflammatory chemicals can be measured in the blood of a person with metabolic syndrome: C-reactive protein, bradykinins, and cytokinins to name a few. Science has discovered that several dread diseases are actually inflammatory in nature (they thrive in an inflammatory environment). Diseases that are known to be fed by inflammatory chemicals include arthritis (joints); gastritis (stomach); Crohn's disease, diverticulitis, and ulcerative colitis (intestines); appendicitis; cirrhosis (liver); numerous cancers; and this book's topic, diabetes.

One of your best defenses against feeding these diseases is to get your body out of its "irritated mood." Acute, temporary inflammation is one of God's healing gifts to the body. Chronic inflammation…well, that's a whole other story.

Do You Still Have Metabolic Syndrome If You're Taking the Appropriate Medication?

During the 20-plus years I've been treating patients, I can't tell you how many times this scenario has occurred during an evaluation:

Mr. Jones, do you personally have any history of cardiovascular or heart disease?
No, I don't.

Do you have high blood pressure?
Not since I've been taking my heart medication.

Have you ever been told you have high cholesterol?
Yes, but the doctor put me on statins. He said that should take care of it.

Have you had your blood sugar checked?
Last year during my annual physical, my doctor told me my sugar was a bit high—so I've been cutting back on desserts.

What about your triglycerides level?
My what?

Medications that help your body metabolize sugar better, control cholesterol, or lower your blood pressure, while helpful, do not *cure* MBS. They act to manage your condition or conditions, not rid your body of them. The best way to change your disease state into a healthy state is to take action against the major culprits in insulin resistance: poor diet and lack of exercise. Over and over again, scientific studies prove that diet modification and exercise have a far better outcome than medication alone.

How Does MBS Begin to Develop?

Researchers have discovered that each of the five markers of MBS stems from the process of insulin resistance. And a frightening fact is, without knowing it, a person can have increased levels of circulating insulin (an early sign of insulin resistance) for *up to 15 years* before they actually become diabetic. That's an awful long time spent driving down the wrong road.

The interrelated subjects of insulin resistance, MBS, prediabetes, and diabetes can be confusing. If you think you may be on the downslope toward diabetes, it's important to be clear on what each term means. The following flowchart describing the role of insulin resistance (IR) in the disease process should help.

IR ➤ **MBS #1: fewer HDLs, more LDLs and triglycerides**
↓
Heart disease, stroke, and so on

IR ➤ **MBS #2: high blood pressure**
↓
Heart failure, kidney damage, and so on

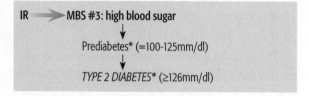

IR ➤ **MBS #3: high blood sugar**
↓
Prediabetes* (=100-125mm/dl)
↓
*TYPE 2 DIABETES** (≥126mm/dl)

IR ➤ **MBS #4: increased clotting**
↓
Associated with blindness, heart attacks, strokes,
amputations, and so on

IR ➤ **MBS #5: heightened inflammation**
↓
Can "fan the flames" of conditions such
as cardiovascular disease, some cancers,
arthritis, and so on

---

* These conditions contribute to many of the diseases discussed in chapter 1.

As you can see, only one of MBS's markers,
elevated blood sugar, can be accurately described
as prediabetes. And in many cases, elevated blood

sugar is the *last* marker to manifest itself. So take a look at these key statements, based on all that we've covered thus far, and understand that you may be in danger even if you have not been diagnosed with high blood sugar:

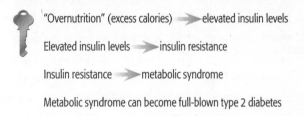

"Overnutrition" (excess calories) ➤ elevated insulin levels

Elevated insulin levels ➤ insulin resistance

Insulin resistance ➤ metabolic syndrome

Metabolic syndrome can become full-blown type 2 diabetes

When Silence Isn't Golden

Why an entire chapter on metabolic syndrome? Simply because MBS sneaks around in your body, setting the stage for some of the most life-threatening diseases you can have. How many of you know someone who died suddenly from a heart attack or stroke, and then it was found that they had cardiovascular disease or diabetes—and didn't even know it?

There is a very real possibility that this silent killer, MBS, is already at work within your body *today*. I want to see this very real threat make you

concerned enough to take action. It's critical to discover where you are *now*. *Now* is the time when you
have the best chance to apply the "health brakes"
and avoid a head-on collision.

In the first part of the next chapter we will focus
on the epidemic of prediabetes. Following that and
continuing in chapter 6 is an easy-to-follow guide to
help you (along with the aid of your physician) get
a real-time handle on your present physical condition, as well as on future health risks.

Chapter 5

Is Diabetes in Your Future?

Lab Tests

B y now you know that diabetes doesn't just "happen" to a person. First you develop insulin resistance; then you will likely acquire one or more traits of metabolic syndrome. Finally, you lose your ability to regulate your blood sugar 'round the clock, and you can head down into *prediabetes*.

While I was researching my previous book, it was the sharp, epidemic-like rise in the prediabetic population that really got my attention. The CDC has calculated that *58 million* Americans presently have prediabetes, or nearly *1 out of every 4* adults over the age of 21. This same study also found that nearly every person discovered to have prediabetes was completely unaware of their problem with sugar management.

If you have the misfortune to be one of the one in four, another study has shown that, over the course of your lifetime, you have an *83 percent chance* of developing diabetes (if you don't make necessary changes).[1] How does it make you feel to know that those 58 million people with prediabetes will soon become 48 million with full-blown diabetes? Could you be one of them?

Who's to Blame?

Genetics seem to get blamed for everything. Unfortunately, they are often guilty as charged. Your unique genetic tendencies may make you lean toward acquiring certain diseases, and such is the case with diabetes and even possibly insulin resistance. Stated even more strongly, according to Drs. Isaacs and Vagnini in their book *Overcoming Metabolic Syndrome,* "genetics determine at what weight you *will* develop insulin resistance, rather than *whether* you will develop it."[2]

That said, just because diabetes runs in your family does not mean you are doomed to get it too. There are *two* factors that must be present for diabetes to develop. The first one you have a great deal of control over. No one gets diabetes without first developing *insulin resistance.* And as we have well established, this is the factor which you can likely do something about.

The second factor, over which you have little control, is that your pancreas must fail to keep up with the demand for higher-than-normal insulin production placed on it. How does a healthy pancreas stop working? Well, it's not a sudden occurrence as in type 1 diabetes, but rather a slow, gradual decline in function.

Recall the process:

1. Eating too much, or eating a steady diet of easily digestible sugar and starches, made insulin overproduction necessary in the first place.

2. Over time your body's insulin receptors (which have spent their days flooded with insulin) began to turn a deaf ear to the "Thou shall store sugar!" commands of all that circulating insulin.

3. In response, your pancreas decided to "yell louder" by making even *more* insulin in hopes that the receptors would "listen" and respond appropriately.

4. Years of excess production of insulin exact a great price from your pancreas. If your pancreas had a tongue, it would be hanging out as it panted and gasped for air! Due to utter exhaustion your pancreas will begin to slow down its insulin production a bit at a time until it gets to the point where it is no longer capable of making enough to maintain your normal blood-sugar level.

Here is where your genetics play a crucial role. *Pancreatic fatigue* is what tends to run in the family. Now, not everyone who becomes insulin-resistant and starts suffering from metabolic syndrome will develop elevated blood sugar (or prediabetes) and progress into full-blown diabetes—but the majority do. However, just because you happen to lack the genetic tendency toward pancreatic fatigue (and therefore full-blown diabetes), this doesn't mean you can ignore the problem of prediabetes and its associated health risks.

Now that you know what you may be up against, your next step is to determine where you lie on the continuum between health and high blood sugar. Then you can construct a plan of action—something I'll help you develop in the rest of this book.

At this point, you need to accurately assess your situation. Do you have any of the markers of metabolic syndrome, and most importantly, have you already acquired the marker that precedes diabetes— elevated blood sugar? This is shown by two bodies of evidence: blood tests and physical measurements. From here through chapter 6 we'll look at what information to obtain and how to interpret the results. So let's get started!

Your Blood Tells Much of the Story

The first place to begin is at your primary-care physician's office. He or she can order or perform your blood work (laboratory testing). However, if you do not have medical insurance coverage and can't afford the expense of going through your doctor, a number of the blood tests I recommend are available by mail order. (See "Resources" at the back of the book for more information.) Some tests may even be available at your local pharmacy.

Blood Test #1: Hemoglobin A1C

The hemoglobin A1C test is often referred to simply as the *A1C test* (pronounced A-one-C). It's the earliest warning an insulin-resistant person can get (apart from a fasting insulin test, which is rarely used outside of research purposes as of this writing).

Remarkably, the A1C test provides you with information regarding the average of your sugar levels *over the past three months!* This is possible because of the amazingly intricate interactions that take place between your red blood cells and the circulating sugars in your bloodstream. Each red blood cell contains four hemoglobin molecules, whose job it is to bind to oxygen molecules and carry them around to your body's cells.

But as some very observant scientists have noted, these hemoglobin molecules also bind to sugar molecules. Because the life span of red blood cells is about three months, the A1C test provides data on just how "sweet" you've been over that period. (Sort of like

Santa, who can tell whether you've been naughty or nice.) The results are given in terms of the *percentage* of hemoglobin A1C molecules that have bound to circulating glucose molecules. The more glucose in your blood, the more binding there will be, and the higher the percentage.

Normal A1C test results lie between 4 and 5.9 percent, although the range may vary slightly among laboratories.[3] "Perfectly normal" is considered by many to be 5 percent. Anywhere between 6 percent and 6.4 percent and you should be concerned—you may very well be prediabetic. Findings such as these indicate that your blood-sugar levels are not well-controlled. And beyond 6.5 to 7.0 percent... unfortunately, you're in diabetes territory. However, even this can be reversible in its earlier stages.

Risk status, disease state	A1C test results
Normal glucose metabolism	4.0% to 5.9%
Elevated—metabolic syndrome likely	6.0% to 6.4%
Diabetes	6.5 to 7.0%

The A1C Test has been historically used within the *known* diabetic population as a method of keeping watch over their sugar management. It is now being used for early identification of prediabetes, though it is still not standard protocol.

Because of its obvious benefit, use of the A1C test has become a growing trend among medical professionals, who are now ordering it as part of the annual blood work for all patients over 21 years old, as well as younger ones who are obese. (Remember that this disease, which used to be called "adult-onset diabetes," affects more and more children and adolescents every year.)

Blood Test #2: *New!*–The GlycoMark Test

A very promising FDA-approved blood test that is gaining much acceptance within the medical community (and even outperforming the A1C test in sensitivity[4]) is the *GlycoMark* test. This test measures what a person's after-meal (postprandial) blood-sugar average is over the previous one to two weeks. As of this writing, the GlycoMark test has not been included in the standard protocol for diagnosis and treatment of MBS and diabetes. But it is my strong belief it will soon become a substitute for the A1C test and gain its place in the blood-sugar-test hall of fame. Just note that this test would likely not be performed along with the A1C test—rather your doctor may use it as a substitute.

Blood Test #3: Fasting Plasma Glucose Test (FPG)

Blood-sugar levels can be measured at any time, but the data that are most telling are from 1) after a period of fasting from food and drink for 12 hours, and 2) two hours following a meal. This first piece of data comes from another "must-have" test, the *fasting plasma glucose,* or *FPG.* As its name indicates, this test provides a measurement of how much glucose (or sugar) is present in your plasma (the fluid portion of your blood) following a period of fasting. Normal FPG level should be less than 100 mg/dl. Anything higher, and a person is said to have *impaired fasting glucose* or IFG.

Blood Test #4: Oral Glucose Tolerance Test (OGTT)

If your doctor finds your sugar level elevated during your office visit, or if your fasting plasma glucose or A1C test comes back higher than normal, then as a follow-up the *oral glucose tolerance test* (OGTT) may be ordered. This test evaluates your body's efficiency at bringing elevated blood-sugar level (the natural result of eating and metabolizing food) back to its normal baseline (less than 100 mg/dl). Two hours following a meal, your pancreas and your body's insulin receptors

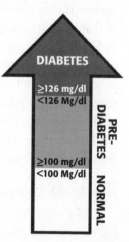

should have managed to bring your sugar levels back down to a near-normal level (100-140 mg/dl). Anything higher and a person is said to have *impaired glucose tolerance,* or IGT.

The OGTT is begun following a fasting period of about eight to ten hours. After an FPG test is performed, you will be given a very sugary, almost syrupy, beverage to drink. Your blood will then be tested hourly for the next three to five hours to determine how well your body processes that sugar out of your bloodstream. Peak sugar levels are measured after one hour, and then your next two blood draws should indicate a decrease, with the final blood draw being in the "normal" range.

More often than not, however, this test is not performed due to the cost and inconvenience to the patient. It is used regularly in the pregnant population as a way of diagnosing and monitoring gestational diabetes. That said, if there seems to be good reason, some physicians do order it for other patients. Typically, before someone's fasting glucose test ever reads positive (even years before), that person will show early signs of insulin resistance (and even prediabetes) in their inability to efficiently process glucose following a meal. And that is what this test is so good at detecting.

Because type 2 diabetes has reached epidemic proportions, the American Diabetes Association has issued the following guidelines, strongly suggesting that medical practitioners order the fasting plasma glucose (FPG) test as well as the oral glucose tolerance test (OGTT) under the following circumstances:

Annual FPG and OGTT recommended for these groups

1. Persons 45 years or older

2. Those who are under 45 years and overweight (body mass index greater than 25)

3. Men or women who have one or more of the following co-conditions:
   - habitually physically inactive
   - parent or sibling who has diabetes
   - member of high-risk ethnic population (for example, African-American, Latino, Native American, Asian-American, Pacific Islander)
   - high-density lipoprotein (HDL) cholesterol less than 35 mg/dl and/or triglyceride level greater than 250 mg/dl
   - hypertensive (blood pressure at or greater than 140/90 mmHg)
   - had impaired glucose tolerance (IGT) or impaired fasting glucose (IFG) on previous testing

- history of vascular disease
- other clinical conditions associated with insulin resistance (for example, dark skin patches)

4. Women who have:
- delivered a baby weighing more than 9 pounds or have been diagnosed with gestational diabetes
- polycystic ovary syndrome

Blood Test #5: Lipid Panel

As discussed in chapter 4, altered lipid profiles (molecule ratios of circulating fats) are one of the components of metabolic syndrome and are most definitely a red flag for eventually developing prediabetes. Elevated levels of LDLs and triglycerides do not bode well for you. Most important, if your levels of HDLs have dropped below 40 mg/dl (for men) or 50 mg/dl (for women), then you've received your season pass to metabolic syndrome. But if you keep on reading and following this book's suggestions, this "season" may well be a short one for you!

In the next chapter we'll round out this self-examination with physical measurements—which are a must in assessing your health risk. Following that, you'll find a summary list of all the tests we've talked about in chapters 5 and 6, so you can be sure to have it in hand when you next visit your doctor.

Chapter 6

Am I at Risk?

Physical Measurements

Just as important as blood tests in determining your risk for metabolic syndrome, prediabetes, or diabetes are the physical measurements or calculations I discuss in this chapter. *Height, weight,* and *blood pressure* are three need-to-know pieces of the puzzle we're assembling. The two other pieces required are measurements of your girth—specifically, your *hip circumference* and *waist circumference.* Progressive doctors may make measurements and calculations in their office, but if not, they're easy to do yourself.

Together with the test results from chapter 5, the three physical findings below will provide you with a crystal-clear picture of your health status and potential risks you face.

Physical Measurement #1: Blood Pressure

This is a quick and easy test that likely everyone has had during their annual routine physical. (If you don't get annual physicals, I do hope reading this

book will change that!) Blood-pressure readings give
your doctor a critically important picture of how well
your heart is working and how much "artery resistance" it must pump against. (If you'd like to keep
an eye on your blood pressure throughout the year,
blood-pressure cuffs, both automated and manual,
can be purchased for home use. Also, many drug-
stores have a self-service blood-pressure cuff located
next to the pharmacy window.) Since we thoroughly
discussed blood pressure in chapter 4, I'll just give
you this quick-reference chart:

Blood Pressure Interpretation	
Low blood pressure	Less than 100 mmHg / 60 mmHg
Normal blood pressure	Less than 120 mmHg / 80 mmHg
Prehypertension	121 to 139 mmHg / 81 to 89 mmHg
High blood pressure (hypertension)	More than 140mmHg / 90 mmHg

Reference Card from the Seventh Report of the Joint National Committee
on Prevention, Detection, Evaluation, and Treatment of High Blood Pressure
(JNC 7), www.nhlbi.nih.gov/guidelines/hypertension/phycard.pdf, accessed 16
September 2009.

Physical Measurement #2: Body Mass Index (BMI)

Actually two measurements rolled into one, *body
mass index,* or *BMI,* is a height-to-weight ratio that
has become an important medical standard for indicating your health risks. Your BMI will place you

in one of four groups: *underweight, normal weight, overweight,* or *obese* (see chart below).

This measurement can be easily performed at home. All you need is to know your present height and your present weight. I emphasize *present* because we adults can shrink over time and our weight certainly fluctuates (in the upward direction, usually). So take the time to make sure you're working with current data.

First you'll need to get an accurate height measurement (not necessarily the one on your driver's license!). This is simple enough. Here's a reliable method my husband uses for tracking our children: Stand with your back against a wall, have someone slide a box (of anything) down the wall above your head until it rests gently against the topmost portion of your skull. Step away so the "box slider" can mark your height with a pencil at the box's bottom edge. Get yourself a tape measure and measure away. Record your height in inches (that is, 61 inches, rather than 5'1").

Next, measure your *body mass,* or weight. Your weight is best measured first thing in the morning, while in your birthday suit. But if you trust your doctor's scale more, go ahead and use that finding if it's recent (deducting two pounds for clothing would be a safe estimate). Record your weight in pounds (not kilograms).

Now plug your measurements into the equation below (a calculator makes quick work of this computation), or use the online Body Mass Index Calculator I have provided on my Web site, **www .RestoringYourTemple.com**. In just a short time you will have new knowledge of an extremely important indicator of your future.

BMI calculation

$$BMI = \left(\frac{\text{Weight in pounds}}{\text{(Height in inches) x (Height in inches)}} \right) \times 703$$

For example, a person who weighs *170 pounds* and is 5 feet 3 inches tall (*63 inches*) will have a BMI of *30.1*. As you'll see from the chart above, that's far too heavy…it's in the obese range.

$$BMI = \left(\frac{\text{170 lbs.}}{\text{(63 inches) x (63 inches)}} \right) \times 703$$

BMI*	Weight status
Below 18.5	Underweight
18.5 to 24.9	Normal
25.0 to 29.9	Overweight
30.0 and above	Obese

* The BMI method does not have individual charts for men and women, or for body-structure type (petite/large frame), hence the ranges indicated.

For those of you who don't want to crunch numbers or go online, I've also provided a reference table on the next page that will give you a pretty good idea of where your BMI lies. Once you know in which weight category your BMI places you, you'll have a much better picture of your present health risk. (Not included is the underweight category, as this is usually not the issue with MBS.)

The Shortcomings of BMI

Muscularly built athletes have bodies that are denser than "normal people" as a result of all those muscles they're carrying around with them. Their BMI will rank too high and will falsely yield a result of "obese," inaccurately suggesting increased health risk.

The elderly, as a result of aging, have *decreased* muscle mass. Their BMI scores will rank them below normal, or "underweight." Again, this may be an inaccurate picture, pointing toward anorexia or body wasting.

Physical Measurement #3: Waist-to-Hip Ratio (WHR)

Researchers have discovered another important measurement for predicting a person's health risk called the *waist-to-hip ratio (WHR)*. Studies have

BMI Table

White=Normal, Gray=Overweight, Dark Gray=Obese

BMI	19	20	21	22	23	24	25	26	27	28	29	30	35	40
Height (in.)							Weight (lbs.)							
58	91	96	100	105	110	115	119	124	129	134	138	143	167	191
59	94	99	104	109	114	119	124	128	133	138	143	148	173	198
60	97	102	107	112	118	123	128	133	138	143	148	153	179	204
61	100	106	111	116	122	127	132	137	143	148	153	158	185	211
62	104	109	115	120	126	131	136	142	147	153	158	164	191	218
63	107	113	118	124	130	135	141	146	152	158	163	169	197	225
64	110	116	122	128	134	140	145	151	157	163	169	174	204	232
65	114	120	126	132	138	144	150	156	162	168	174	180	210	240
66	118	124	130	136	142	148	155	161	167	173	179	186	216	247
67	121	127	134	140	146	153	159	166	172	178	185	191	223	255
68	125	131	138	144	151	158	164	171	177	184	190	197	230	262
69	128	135	142	149	155	162	169	176	182	189	196	203	236	270
70	132	139	146	153	160	167	174	181	188	195	202	207	243	278
71	136	143	150	157	165	172	179	186	193	200	208	215	250	286
72	140	147	154	162	169	177	184	191	199	206	213	221	258	294
73	144	151	159	166	174	182	189	197	204	212	219	227	265	302
74	148	155	163	171	179	186	194	202	210	218	225	233	272	311
75	152	160	168	176	184	192	200	208	216	224	232	240	279	319
76	156	164	172	180	189	197	205	213	221	230	238	246	287	328

Partnership for Healthy Weight Management, Body Mass Index (BMI), www.consumer.gov/weightloss/bmi.htm, accessed June 5, 2009.

shown it to be a better indicator of type 2 diabetes in men than the BMI.[1] And still other research has found it to be a more accurate measure of obesity in the elderly population.[2] If you are going to understand your risk for prediabetes or diabetes, then you'll want to add this scientifically proven method also.

You may have heard people's body types described as "apple-shaped" or "pear-shaped." (I love the picture this conjures up in describing where a person tends to carry extra body weight.) An undeniable increased health risk has been associated with those who have "apple-shaped" bodies—those whose fat is collected around their bellies. Conversely, "pear-shaped" individuals, who have a relatively trim stomach yet sport big hips and too much "junk in their trunk," are deemed luckier than their apple counterparts. Although you pear-shaped individuals have likely never felt "lucky" about your shape when in the fitting room, in the health world you are most certainly blessed!

So what does fruit and body shape have to do with diabetes? Scientific research indicates that stern health warnings are in order for individuals whose waist measurement alone is "over the top"—even before their waist dimension is compared with their hips. These waist circumferences pose *very high health risks* (including diabetes) to the individuals who have them:

 Men: Waist circumference of 40 inches (101cm) or more

Women: Waist circumference of 35 inches (89cm) or more

You can easily measure yourself with a flexible measuring tape. Wrap it around your midsection at the height of your belly button, starting and ending at the exact same point. Note the number in inches, as we will use in a moment to calculate your waist-hip ratio.

Okay, so where exactly are your hips? I'm sure I'd lose some of you if I described where your *actual* hips lie from the viewpoint of a physical therapist, so for the purpose of this measurement simply wrap the tape measure around the broadest point of your hips, or pelvis. Once again, begin and end at the exact same point.

Now plug both measurements (in inches) into the equation below. Then look at the chart and see where you land: low, moderate, or high risk. For some of you this simple home exercise will be an immediate wakeup call.

WHR = waist circumference ÷ hip circumference

For example: If your waist circumference = *40 inches* and your hip circumference = *38 inches,* then your waist-to-hip ratio equals 40 ÷ 38, or = *1.05.* With that result, you would be knee-deep in risk!

Waist-to-Hip Ratio Chart

Male	Female	Health risk based solely on WHR
0.95 or below	0.80 or below	Low
0.96 to 1.0	0.81 to 0.85	Moderate
1.0 or more	0.85 or more	High

Not all diabetics or prediabetics are overweight (with elevated BMIs and WHRs). You may just be one of those people who look physically fit on the outside but are health-challenged on the inside. Beating this high blood-sugar thing and its associated risks requires you to look at yourself through many different windows. If the view through any of those windows doesn't fit the picture of good health, *it's time to act.*

At this stage, here's the next key step. Now that you're armed with knowledge of your potential health risks, make an appointment to see your primary-care physician. Specifically ask your doctor to order some of the blood tests we discussed in chapter 5 (ones you haven't had performed within the last year). You can us the checklist on page 89. Make sure you write down your blood pressure reading and your weight and height stats (and any circumference measurements that are taken). When your blood-test results come back—even if they are normal—ask for a copy. You may want to use it for comparison as the years go on.

Second, turn to the next chapter so you can learn how to turn over a new leaf and help your body become your lifelong friend, rather than an antagonist. What you'll learn there can make a powerful change in your health!

Here's a checklist you can copy and take to your next doctor's visit. You can also download it from my Web site, www.RestoringYourTemple.com.

Blood Tests

- Hemoglobin A1C (or GlycoMark)
- Fasting Plasma Glucose Tolerance (FPG)
- Oral Glucose Tolerance Test (OGTT)
- Lipid Profile:
    Total cholesterol
    HDL
    LDL
    Triglycerides

Physical Tests

- Blood pressure
- Height and weight (BMI)
- Waist and hip circumference (WHR)

Chapter 7

Marshmallows for Dinner

What You Don't Know About the Food You Eat

Who would actually eat *marshmallows* for dinner—besides an unsupervised four-year old? Actually, in a very real way I used to do just that—and likely you do as well. Let me explain. Marshmallows are little cylinders of puffed-up fructose and sucrose. They land in your stomach like mini sugar bombs, poised to make your blood sugar blast up like a rocket.

Well, what I learned that came as a real surprise to me is that all simple carbohydrates (refined starches such as white rice, pasta, potatoes, and white bread) "go down" like marshmallows and make your blood glucose shoot up in a Mt. Vesuvius surge. And very little digestion is needed for this to occur. Often, before these foods even reach your stomach, the saliva in your mouth has partially broken them down into pure sugar molecules. And this sends your blood-sugar level soaring just as if you were eating marshmallows!

So the next time you're sitting at the table, picture that pile of white rice sitting on your dinner plate, or the helping of potatoes you just served yourself, as nothing but a mound of mini marshmallows. Not so appetizing or innocent anymore, huh? I have painted this word picture many times for my patients and friends, and that image alone has been enough to convince many of them to seek healthier alternatives. I know it keeps me from making poor food choices almost every day.

By now you know you need to avoid excessive sugar spikes because they will eventually lead to insulin resistance and then push you downhill toward all sorts of maladies. There's a lot at stake.

The next step is to learn to eat in a way that keeps your blood sugar as even-keeled as possible. Blood sugar will *always* rise after eating—this is natural and normal. But you can work to temper that rise by learning *what* and *when* to eat, as well as knowing how to partner foods with one another for the best outcome: a moderate, short-term upward rise in blood glucose. With this knowledge, you'll be able to make better decisions about food choices, which will improve your body's ability to metabolize sugar.

That said, this chapter is not meant to be a complete dietary guide. Rather, it shines a spotlight on hidden danger areas within your diet...where a little change on your part will make a *huge* difference in your blood sugar.

Not All Carbohydrates Are Created Equal

All carbohydrates ("carbs") are comprised of sugar molecules. When digested, carbs yield energy the most quickly of any food source because they are converted into glucose molecules without much ado.

- *Simple carbohydrates* common to our diet include table sugar (sucrose), fruit-based sugar (fructose), brewed beverage sugar (maltose), and milk-based sugar (lactose).

- *Complex carbohydrates,* or starches, which include items such as bread, rice, pasta, and potatoes, are made up of sugar molecules that are linked together in a chainlike fashion. In their natural state, most sources of complex carbohydrates are loaded with fiber.

- A subset group of complex carbohydrates— which act similarly to simple carbohydrates—are *refined carbohydrates.* Refined carbs are made from *processed* grain that has been stripped of its bran and thus a large part of its fiber and nutrition. The more refined a carbohydrate is, or the less encumbered with fiber, the more quickly it breaks down into simple sugar molecules. White rice, refined flour, and regular pasta are modern-day examples of such foods.

If you want to place the blame for the rising rate of diabetes in our country on something, you could blame it on our taste buds! In the early 1900s we began to develop an appetite for products made with refined flour. Before that time *the entire grain* of wheat was roughly ground by stone mills, bran and all. The resulting brown and somewhat rough-textured flour was all that was available to the average person for baking and pasta-making.

When technology made it possible to separate the outer bran from the inner pulp in a grain of wheat on a large scale, much nutritional value and protection from disease was thrown out with the bran! The introduction of steel rollers into grain mills at about the same time also enabled the flour to be ground into a fine powder. And thus began our love affair with white, fluffy, nutritionally starved breads, cakes, and cookies. And quite quickly, potbellied stoves gave way to potbellied people.

To better aid your meal selection of carbohydrates, I've compiled two lists of foods below. The first includes carbs that are best avoided altogether—or at least kept to occasional guest appearances. While this list is not exhaustive, it covers the starchy food items most Americans eat without ever thinking they might be consuming marshmallows in disguise!

Carbohydrates You'd Do Better to Avoid (or Limit Significantly)

White bread: sliced, bagels, Italian bread, dinner rolls, biscuits, hot dog and hamburger rolls

White rice

White, Yukon gold, red potatoes

White pasta: all shapes and sizes, including noodles

White sugar...really, *all* sugar needs to be limited

Fruit juice

Soft drinks

Beer, wine, and liquors

Usually the less processing a food undergoes (the more it looks like its natural state), the better it is for you. Plain and simple, a diet high in fiber is good for your sugar control. The more fiber a carbohydrate food contains, the more slowly its sugar is released into your bloodstream, which lowers the resulting peak in your blood sugar. *It's a good thing!* as Martha Stewart would say. Speaking of good things, below is a list that gives you better, blood-sugar-stabilizing carbohydrate options to choose from.

Healthier Carbohydrate Options

Whole-grain breads

Brown rice

Sweet potatoes

Whole-grain or low-glycemic-index* pasta (for example,
Dreamfields)
Honey
Whole fruit instead of juice (for example, apple, orange)
Fruit juice diluted with 4 parts sparkling water (a great substi-
tute for soda pop)
* See sidebar on next page

How to Keep a Lid on Your Sugar Spikes

We've exposed the dangers that certain forms of
carbohydrates can pose to your sugar metabolism.
But carbs are not the only thing we eat! Other compounds such as proteins and fats and food groups
such as fruits and vegetables have their own unique
effects. In order to accurately gauge their individual
effect on the rise of glucose levels, scientists came
up with two scales of measurement.

Used today in the field of nutrition and diabetes
management are *glycemic index* and the *glycemic load*
(see sidebars). Their findings agree for the most part,
but results do vary greatly for a few food items—
particularly those containing high sugar content
along with high fiber (for example, watermelon,
cantaloupe). While glycemic index has been more
widely publicized, glycemic load is said to be a more
accurate measurement of a food's real-time effect
on the body.

Either way these studies have proven invaluable. We now know that most vegetables have little effect on blood sugar; most fruits (and all fruit juices) produce sugar spikes when eaten separately; and fats, proteins, and complex (unrefined) carbs take a long time to digest—which is a good thing.

The Glycemic Index

Created in 1981 by Drs. David Jenkins and M.S. Wolever, this index indicates the effect that eating a food containing 50 grams of carbohydrates would have on a person's blood sugar. Pure glucose was used as the baseline and assigned a "100" on the glycemic scale. (This happens to be identical to the effect of a slice of white bread.) Foods whose glycemic index scores below 55 are considered great, those scoring 56 to 69 are to be eaten in moderation, and foods scoring above 70 are to be avoided altogether or limited in quantity and frequency.[1]

The Glycemic Load

In 1997, researchers at Harvard University introduced the concept of *glycemic load,* which takes into account not only the *amount* of a food, but also its *fiber content* (which, as you are now aware, slows the breakdown of a carbohydrate into sugar). The glycemic load is calculated by dividing the glycemic index of a food by the number of grams of carbs in a serving of that food. The lower the load, the better choice a food is for people with insulin resistance. Glycemic load is considered low when scoring below 10 and moderate between 11 and 20. If greater than 20, it is recommended that the food be avoided altogether by those with metabolic syndrome.[2]

Some Foods Make Great Partners

Pairing foods with protein. In their book *The Insulin-Resistant Diet,* Drs. Cheryle Hart and Mary Kay Grossman suggest that the best way to regulate blood sugar is to always eat a protein as part of every meal and snack.[3] Proteins digest slowly, give the body a prolonged feeling of satiation (fullness), and can be a low-fat source of fuel. So even when eating good choices such as a piece of fruit or a few whole-grain crackers, pairing those foods with protein will even out your blood sugar much better than if they were eaten alone (even if it raises the calorie count). Myself, I sometimes snack on just a protein—for example, a handful of nuts—and find it seems to hold off my hunger quite well. (At the end of this chapter I've listed my own personal application of this principle in the form of meal and snack suggestions.)

Partnering proteins and carbs. Again in an effort to slow digestion, Doctors Hart and Grossman also advocate partnering equal servings of protein with carbohydrates.[4] For example, for every one serving of meat, you can have one serving of rice. Or if you have two servings of a carbohydrate (for example, bread), then you'll need to partner it with two servings of protein, such as eggs. In this way the speed at which carbs are broken down can be buffered by the slowness of protein digestion. The overall effect is a moderate, "doable" rise in sugar.

Partnering fats and carbs. Much to my surprise (and joy), in *The South Beach Diet Supercharged*, cardiologist Arthur Agatston recommends partnering carbs with *healthy* fats to slow down the digestion process of the carbohydrate. Why am I so happy about this? Discovering that it's better for my blood sugar when my half a bagel is smeared with a bit of reduced fat cream cheese or that my piece of bread at a restaurant is better for me if dipped in olive oil has increased the yumminess factor of those carbs many times over. No more dry bread or toast for me—yahoo!

Vegetables (many of which are carbs) are freebies in these two methods of food partnering, meaning that you may eat as much as you'd like of *most* vegetables without experiencing an unbalanced effect on your blood-sugar metabolism. I say *most* because in Dr. Agatston's book (*The South Beach Diet Supercharged* or the original *South Beach Diet*) you'll discover that corn, beets, carrots, and sweet peas are exceptions. These veggies contain an extremely high amount of sugar!

Time Out for Your Pancreas

In 2005, when Dr. Agatston's book *The South Beach Diet* first hit the market, I, like many in the health field, rolled my eyes at the publishing of yet another "diet book." That is—before I had a chance to read it. What I found upon closer investigation was not just another weight-loss plan, but rather a clever way to recalibrate sugar metabolism, restore circulating lipid balance, and better yet, reset the sensitivity of the body's insulin receptors! The final outcome, along with potentially permanent weight loss, is a maintainable approach to eating that doesn't leave a person feeling like they're stuck on a "diet."

What sets Dr. Agatston's method apart is his prescription of an initial two-week "pancreas rest and insulin receptor resensitization" protocol.[7] Although I highly recommend that you read his book for yourself (see "Resources" at the end of this book), let me attempt to explain the concept in a nutshell. I'm sure you'll see how much sense it makes, given all you now know about blood-sugar metabolism.

Because blood-sugar spikes occur when simple sugars (such as sucrose, fructose, and maltose) are introduced to the body, followed by insulin flooding, Dr. Agatston recommends a drastic approach. (Yes, out-of-control blood sugar demands drastic action!) This method calls for no sugar, no carbs—breads, beer, fruit, fruit juices, anything—for the first two weeks! You make all your meals and snacks solely from healthy, lean proteins and vegetables (minus those on his "not-so-good" list, as mentioned above).

Agatston's research review and patient studies have shown remarkable improvements in blood chemistry in those who endure those first two weeks and also continue to eat a health-modified diet going forward. This two-week vacation from sugar spikes and insulin flooding is like abstaining from using perfume or cologne for a while so your nose can regain its sensitivity to smells once again. Then a moderate amount of fragrance can be slowly reintroduced and enjoyed again.

An Easy Eating Plan

If you're having trouble putting all this information into a plan of action, don't worry. Below you will find a week of mealtime menu suggestions which I often use at home when cooking for myself or for my family. Use them in good health!

A week of *breakfast* suggestions

1. High fiber, low-sugar cereal, 1 percent milk, ½ cup blueberries

2. One slice whole-grain toast (buttered lightly with butter/canola oil spread), 1-2 scrambled eggs

3. Steel-cut oatmeal topped with milk, walnuts, cinnamon, and a bit of brown sugar

4. Egg-white omelet with diced tomatoes and low-fat cheese, turkey bacon

5. Low-fat cottage cheese, ½ banana, sliced almonds, drizzle of honey

6. Fried eggs (in olive oil), Canadian bacon

7. Yogurt (low-sugar), chopped strawberries, ¼ cup granola

A week of *lunch* suggestions

1. Sandwich (half or whole): Turkey lunch meat, low-fat Swiss cheese, mustard

2. Tuna salad with chopped celery, peppers, onion, dressed with lemon juice and olive oil, salt and pepper, or light mayonnaise, served over a bed of salad greens

3. Chicken breast meat, sliced tomatoes, low glycemic pasta salad

4. Tomato soup (made with 1 percent milk), ½ melted cheese sandwich (reduced-fat cheddar or Swiss)

5. Black bean soup with dollop of low-fat sour cream

6. Chef salad topped with ham, chopped hard-cooked egg, tomatoes, and a bit of blue cheese (a little goes a long way in flavor)

7. Ham and cheese between two romaine lettuce leaves (instead of bread), carrot sticks with dip

A week of *dinner* suggestions

1. Baked chicken, brown rice with low-fat gravy (use sparingly), and steamed carrots

2. Low-glycemic pasta with tomato sauce and meatballs (lean beef, or pork and beef mix)

3. Homemade chicken and vegetable soup, one high-fiber or low-glycemic dinner roll

4. Turkey chili topped with low-fat shredded cheddar cheese

5. Specialty chicken sausage (for instance, with broccoli rabe and roasted tomatoes), baked sweet potato, broccoli

6. Lean beef burger (no bun), tomato salad, grilled zucchini

7. Pork roast, cauliflower, broccoli, and carrot medley, packaged brown rice pilaf

Condiments with a Cure

Spice is nice. Spicy foods digest more slowly than mild-mannered ones, so add some heat if you can stomach it!

Cinnamon. Half a teaspoon of cinnamon a day has been shown to lower blood sugar. It has the added advantage of being a wonderful antioxidant (a cancer-fighting chemical).[5]

Apple cider vinegar. When two tablespoons are mixed with a glass of water and drunk before a meal, studies have shown this helps to lower postmeal blood-sugar highs.[6]

Honey. This natural sweetener has a lower glycemic index than table sugar and has been shown to strengthen the immune system as well.

Snacks That Keep Your Blood Sugar Steady

Thus far we have talked solely about keeping your sugar from spiking. But we also need to address dips in sugar levels, which could sabotage your best efforts. The best way to keep your blood sugar steady on the high end of the spectrum is to take care not to let it drop too *low*. A below-normal blood-sugar level will almost certainly send you on a "carb hunt"— looking for an immediate sugar fix in between meals.

And even if you are able to fight back those cravings, you will likely show up to your next meal ravenous and consequently eat many more calories than you should.

My patients frequently ask me what *I* eat when I get hungry between meals. Well, having learned from the above guidelines for healthy eating, I have some favorite "go-to" snacks, which I eat midmorning and again in the midafternoon. Most times I grab one of the following:*

- Half an avocado, a teaspoon of blue cheese dressing, black pepper
- A handful of almonds, cashews, or walnuts
- About two dozen pistachios
- A low-fat cheese stick
- A carrot, apple, or half a banana with a tablespoon of peanut, almond, or cashew butter
- A small low-sugar organic fruit yogurt topped with cinnamon (Greek yogurts have twice the protein of traditional yogurt)
- Low-fat cottage cheese with honey and cinnamon, topped with berries or banana slices
- Hummus, either with cucumber or sweet pepper slices, or with five or six baked pita chips

---

* Everyone needs to be allowed to eat a cookie or a handful of chips occasionally—I am not suggesting an inflexible approach to eating.

- A small piece of dark chocolate
- A mini bag of microwave popcorn (a variety with no trans fats)

Congratulations on taking the first big step toward your recovery from insulin resistance—educating yourself on the dietary basics needed to achieve improved blood-sugar metabolism.

I hope this information has revealed a whole new aspect of food basics to you and that it will help you look at the food you put in your mouth in a whole different light. These days I am viewing sugars and refined carbs as harmful, not helpful—as *trouble* rather than a treat. I hope you're beginning to think this way too.

Chapter 8

More Than Enough

Figuring Out How to Take a Healthy Portion

Pairing and partnering foods appropriately, which we discussed in the previous chapter, will do wonders in helping to regulate your blood sugar. However, regularly eating too much of *anything* is going to stress out your pancreas and create "deafness" in your insulin receptors. In addition to making poor food choices, most people struggling with poor sugar metabolism are overweight and underexercised. Nobody sets out in life determined to get fat (except maybe sumo wrestlers). But regardless of intentions, many in our country have become just that.

Frighteningly, the obesity epidemic in America makes the diabetes epidemic look mild. *Two out of every three people in the United States today are overweight.* If you're carrying around an "extra helping of you," especially in your belly area, then I suspect you are insulin-resistant right now. Belly fat has been found to be more harmful than a whole "trunk

load" of extra padding, as we discussed in chapter
6. Apple-shaped people are at a much higher health
risk than pear-shaped ones.

When "fat happens," there is typically only one
cause: You have eaten more calories than your body
has needed for fuel. This overnourishment is also
responsible for excessive sugar loads, which, as I've
said before, eventually produces insulin resistance
and its entire brotherhood of disease. This happens
regardless of whether your weight gain came from
eating too much ice cream and potato chips (bad
stuff) or too much baked chicken and brown rice
(good stuff).

When we carry around too much weight, it begins
to have toxic effects on our body's organs and systems.
According to researcher Michèle Guerre-Millo,

> Our understanding of the relation between
> obesity and metabolic risk factors is growing
> rapidly. This understanding is based on the
> discovery of multiple products released
> from adipocytes [fat cells]. In the presence
> of obesity, these products are released in
> abnormal amounts. Each of these products
> has been implicated in the causation of one
> or another of the metabolic risk factors.[1]

In other words, when the fat cells in your body
become overstuffed as a result of overeating and poor
sugar metabolism, they actually feed back into the

problem of metabolic syndrome (MBS) by releasing health-jeopardizing substances that wreak havoc on your anatomy. High amounts of circulating fat molecules (blood-borne lipids) have been shown to cause your liver to release harmful hormones into your body as well. In other words, the cells of a body in a "fat state" release bad chemicals into your bloodstream, further eroding your health.

Correcting Portion Distortion

Diet and weight-loss programs are big business in the U.S., grossing billions of dollars annually, because we as a nation eat too much. In my earlier book *Overcoming Overeating* I included some of the following information on the subject of portion control, along with some very useful tips on how to make portion control a part of your life.[2]

Researcher and registered dietician Jim Painter, PhD, RD, says that "most of us eat whatever's on our plate." In one study he conducted, people who unknowingly ate soup out of self-refilling bowls consumed 73 percent more than those who were given regular bowls. "They just wanted to get to the bottom,"[3] he remarked. Another study by Painter's research group showed that people who ate ice cream out of larger bowls with larger spoons ate a far greater amount than those who ate out of smaller-sized bowls with smaller spoons.[4]

Portion size is so important that it appears to trump even food *type*. In his documentary "Portion Size Me," Painter placed two of his students on a 30-day fast-food "diet." Eating only what was given to them (proper portion sizes), both students actually lost weight! Now, I'm *not* validating continual fast-food consumption as a part of a healthy lifestyle. But I think Dr. Painter's findings drive home the point: Weight loss and maintenance are tied directly into portion control.

Because, as we've seen, too much of a good thing can become a bad thing, here are some tips to improve your portion control:

1. When serving yourself, take a smaller amount than usual, and then put away the leftovers *before* you begin to eat. (It's risky to bring the extra to the table—remember, it takes 20 minutes for your brain to get the message that your hunger has been satisfied.)

2. Know visually what a healthy-sized portion should look like:

    - A one-cup serving of rice or mashed potatoes = the size of a tennis ball
    - One portion of meat = the size of your palm and approximately the thickness of your index finger
    - A serving of vegetables fits inside your two cupped hands

- One serving of fruit = the size of your fist, and so on...

3. Don't eat out of containers. You have no idea how much you are eating, and the temptation to overeat is nearly overpowering!

4. Check the label for portion sizes and calorie counts when eating prepared, prepackaged foods.

5. When ordering in a restaurant:

   - Send the bread basket back! If you love bread (or are famished), take a small piece of bread with some butter or better yet, olive oil, and *then* send the rest of it away. (Adding the fat here in moderation satisfies your hunger more and controls your blood sugar better than bread alone.)

   - Eat only half of your meal and doggie-bag the rest. (If you doubt your ability to stop halfway through, ask your waiter to package half of it *before* you begin.)

   - Order an appetizer and a salad instead of an entree.

   - If you absolutely must indulge in a dessert, share it.

Keeping portion size under control is a major strategy in avoiding excessive sugar spikes, which lead to insulin resistance and the sugar-metabolism problems we seek to steer clear of. In due time, less on your plate will mean less of *you*. And that will do wonders for your blood profile (not to mention your body profile!).

Now that you've learned how food *quality* and food *quantity* can have damaging or healing effects on your blood-sugar metabolism, it's time to act on what you know. Take baby steps, or jump in with both feet. In either case you will be better off than yesterday, and tomorrow you'll be better off than you are today. Every day, and at every meal, you have the opportunity to impact your life…by eating to pursue more good years, or to inherit fewer, not-so-good years. I pray you choose the first.

Chapter 9

"Ex"-Rated

*"Ex"-ercise—a Necessity If You're
Serious About Preventing Diabetes*

If we were face-to-face, several of you would likely inform me that you *absolutely hate* to exercise. I hear you. As a physical therapist I've listened to that same complaint countless times over the last 20 years or so. For those of you who view *exercise* as a dirty word, let me say from the get-go that you are not alone.

Truth be told, some days I've heard a bit of "I hate exercising" whining coming from my own mouth! Strange—since I used to be a very competitive athlete in my younger years. As a teenager I played softball, field hockey, volleyball, and was a county-ranked sprinter on my high-school track team. In college, I had to replace team sports with aerobic-type classes and weight lifting. During my two pregnancies and throughout my children's pre-school and elementary school years I mixed up my exercise routine quite a bit—from gym-based exercise to "going it on my own." Back then, staying active and in shape came easily to me. I truly enjoyed all types of exercise, and it provided a much-needed "mommy-time" break.

Well, fast-forward into my forties (the decade of decline for many). I still enjoy exercising...well, most of the time. The problem is that my days have become much fuller with writing projects and deadlines, teaching college students, treating patients, raising two teenagers, and partnering with my husband in church ministry. Now there are more days when I either don't feel like doing it or I really can't "afford" the time.

You may be at a similar place in life. When that sort of resistance arises, what do you do? It helps me to try to keep my mind focused on the purpose—better health. This requires an *intentional* change in perspective. Rather than feeling the weight of "having to exercise," I look at it this way: I have the *ability* and the *means* to stay physically active. It is a gift I've been given, and it's a gift I want to pass on to myself and those I love. If you think of exercise like this, you're more likely to see it as a privilege than as a punishment—which does wonders for your follow-through in actually doing it!

All exercise is beneficial when it comes to diabetes prevention. In this chapter, I would love to see you become thoroughly convinced of your urgent need to become physically active on a regular basis—in whatever way, shape, or form you choose. Some of you will find you are better at staying on a planned-out exercise program. Or like me, you'll find you lean more toward variety. I enjoy biking, walking, playing tennis, and performing various strength and flexibility exercises—and occasionally I get to enjoy paddling around in my family's two-man kayak with my husband. Today, as you can see, my program is not much of "a program" at all. Yet I make an effort to remain physically active every day, and I strive to spend three days a week "moving on purpose" for 30 to 90 minutes (depending on the activity). Most weeks I succeed, but when I don't, I'm careful not to pile a load of guilt on myself, which is counterproductive. I just try to do better the following week.

The important thing isn't *how* you exercise, but that you *do* exercise. I hope you'll intentionally become a "mover and a shaker"—and then, as the months pass by, you may find there is less of you that shakes!

Exercise Can Slow, Halt, or Reverse the Process of Diabetes

For those who are facing the very real possibility of metabolic syndrome, prediabetes, or diabetes, exercise must be viewed as *a matter of life and death.* Does that sound awfully dramatic? Studies show

that a full 83 percent of persons with prediabetes
will eventually become diabetic if their lifestyles
remain unchanged!

If you are indeed prediabetic, regular exercise
has been shown to decrease your possibility (or more
accurately, probability) of becoming diabetic by *18
to 20 percent*.[1] And even if you eventually move into
full-blown diabetes (as 65 percent of prediabetics
will), that same study found that those prediabetics
who lose weight and increase their physical activity
can actually *delay* the development of type 2 diabetes
by an average of 11 years. That's a major benefit from
"getting a move on"!

Suppose you've been identified as prediabetic and
have begun taking prescription medication. Do you
get a "pass" with the exercise thing? In a word—no.
Medication is not nearly as effective in protecting
your health as lifestyle changes are. When compared
to weight loss and exercise, preventive medication
has been shown to delay the onset of type 2 diabetes
by an average of only 3 years. Compare that with
the impressive *11-year delay* mentioned above and
achieved solely with diet and exercise. (Add diet and
exercise to medication, and who knows how long
you could keep diabetes at bay?) No matter which
way you look at it, studies confirm that you are
better able to avoid, delay, or even reverse diabetes
by becoming more physically active.

Now, if your test results reveal you *don't* have prediabetes, please don't wait until you do before you begin to "move on purpose." Steer clear of MBS by supercharging your healthy eating approach and by keeping your body in shape and losing some weight. Increased physical activity results in a win-win situation for everyone who can do it.

What If You're Already Diabetic?

Even if you've been diagnosed with full-blown, medically treated diabetes, modification of your lifestyle with diet and exercise holds much benefit. Regular physical activity can enable you to bring your elevated sugar levels under better control, which may lead to your needing less medication. It may also prevent you from becoming insulin-dependent, and thus having to administer daily injections to yourself. And who knows, some of you who are newly diagnosed may even be able to revert to the prediabetic, even the pre-prediabetic stage—with lowered A1C and normal fasting blood sugar results!

If your doctor has cleared you to safely exercise—do it. I have a friend who, by weight loss and exercise, was able to reverse her diabetes diagnosis (along with the MBS factors) and come off not only her diabetes medication, but also her cholesterol and high-blood-pressure medications—all in less than a year! I hope that is true for you!

How Exercise Impacts Sugar Metabolism

Whenever I give my patients a home exercise program, I find they're much better at follow-through when I take the time to explain *why* they're performing a particular exercise and *how it fits* into their overall recovery plan. Let's take the same approach here.

Insulin resistance, as you now well know, is the villain. We spent the last two chapters looking at what, how, and how much to eat to protect ourselves from excessive insulin flooding into our bloodstream.

However, controlling sugar spikes addresses only part of the problem. As you recall from chapter 3, the other issue leading to MBS takes place within the insulin receptors themselves—over time, due to repeated insulin floods, they become resistant to the body's own insulin.

I have recently discovered that physical activity can play a major role in addressing this second part of insulin resistance. And because I am a physical therapist, I find the wonderfully beneficial role exercise plays in regulating sugar metabolism especially exciting!

Increased Sensitivity of Insulin Receptors

Insulin receptors act much like a padlock on a cell's "storage shed." That padlock can be unlocked by only one key, the hormone insulin. The primary sugar storage cells that the insulin "key" unlocks are found in the liver and the body's skeletal muscles and fat. After insulin receptors become desensitized, many remain in a "locked position," leaving all those excessive circulating glucose molecules with nowhere to go. So round and round they flow within your bloodstream. Naturally, this faulty sugar-storage system results in elevated blood-sugar levels.

Scientific research has discovered an effective way to improve the sensitivity of insulin receptor sites in the skeletal muscles—exercise! How exactly does this work? Well, many researchers are asking that same question. One puts it this way after yet another failed attempt to uncover the mechanism behind the "why":

> Although the post-exercise increase in muscle insulin sensitivity has been characterized [documented] in considerable detail, the basic mechanisms underlying this phenomenon remain a mystery.[2]

So even though we presently do not know the *why,* we do know the *what:* Exercise increases the body's sensitivity to insulin. Now there's one great reason to exercise. But wait, there's more...

Weight Loss

Another benefit of increased physical activity is *weight loss*—something that's on people's minds quite a lot of the time. It's a simple principle—the more you move, the more calories you'll burn. Muscles, heart, and lungs that are working harder require more food (sugar). The more intense your activity is, the more sugar molecules you'll "burn through" as fuel. And not just at the time of exercise. Studies have shown that your metabolic rate remains elevated for about one hour following your exercise session. So even while you are cooling down, your calories are burning up!

Further, exercised muscles grow in size to meet the demand placed on them. The more muscle mass (volume) you gain, the more calories you will burn, because muscle burns more calories than fat does (even when you are just sitting around). In the chart below you'll find examples of typical forms of exercise and the approximate number of calories you can expect to burn in a period of 30 minutes. As noted, the actual number of calories burned depends on your body weight. (A larger body requires more energy to move and needs a greater supply of the body's resources to function.) Seeing this in black and white sure can make eating a couple of 100-calorie cookies not worth the effort it will take to burn them off!

Calories Burned During 30 Minutes of Exercise

Activity / Individual's weight	120 lbs	140 lbs	160 lbs	180 lbs
Aerobics	222	258	294	333
Basketball	225	264	300	339
Cycling (10 mph)	165	192	219	246
Golf (pulling clubs)	138	162	186	210
Hiking	135	156	180	201
Jogging	279	324	372	417
Skating (ice and roller)	177	207	237	264
Skiing (snow and water)	171	198	228	255
Swimming (moderate pace)	239	270	309	348
Tennis	180	207	237	267
Walking	195	228	261	291
Weight training	198	228	261	294

Positive Health Steps, "Calories burned per activity chart," http://positivehealth steps.com/calories-burned.shtml, accessed October 5, 2009.

Improved Cardiovascular Health

Any physical activity that causes you to breathe more deeply and more frequently will, in time, increase the capacity of your heart and lungs to pump blood and oxygen around your body. This

enables your circulatory and respiratory systems to
better meet the demands placed on them. And there
are even greater benefits. Exercise-induced gains in
these two body systems have been shown to lower
blood pressure and positively affect lipid balance
("up with the good cholesterol, down with the bad").
If you're facing metabolic syndrome, these are fine
bonuses!

Improved Strength (and Flexibility)

Increased physical activity can improve both the
strength and flexibility of your skeletal muscles. In
the heading, I placed "flexibility" in parentheses
because I don't want to imply that increased muscle
flexibility has an impact on sugar metabolism. That
said, restoring and maintaining muscle extensibility
is nonetheless a basic component of overall physical
wellness. In fact, it is vital to restoring and maintaining joint and muscle health.

On the other hand, increasing your physical
strength, and thus the overall weight (mass) of your
muscles, greatly improves your sugar metabolism!
As I noted before, muscle tissue burns more calories than fat. Sporting bigger muscles enables you
to use up more of the calories you eat (feeding those
hungry muscles), which leaves less sugar floating
around in need of storage.

Some basic observations: Muscle strength can

be gained by lifting and lowering weights using free weights or Universal or Nautilus–type systems. It can also be obtained by lifting and lowering your body against gravity (floor exercises, Pilates). In addition, strength gains can be achieved by using resistance-type training: pulling against exercise tubing or bending Bowflex-type bars or cables. Whatever resistance weight training method you choose, your body will thank you for putting it through all that trouble.

Other advantages of strength training beyond the benefit of increased metabolic rate are that you'll be less susceptible to injury and more capable of performing challenging activities. Also, your bones will hold onto their calcium better—which can work to prevent or slow the progression of osteoarthritis and osteoporosis. In fact, this has helped many of my postmenopausal patients whose bone scans revealed demineralization of their bones (osteopenia or osteoporosis). These women have shown marked improvement in their bone density as a result of incorporating strength training or weight-bearing exercise (for example, walking) into their weekly routines.

Where to Begin?

Don't have a clue about stretching or strengthening your muscles? In my book *Overcoming Back and Neck Pain,* I detail the most important stretches to perform when trying to heal from, or avoid, back and neck pain. Each stretching exercise is accompanied by an illustration of the muscle to be stretched as well as a photo of the stretch itself.

And how about strength training? Afraid you might hurt yourself if you join a gym? In the same book, you can find carefully chosen beginner-to-moderate-level strength training exercises also. And if you suffer from spine-related pain that has prevented you from exercising, do yourself a favor and pick up that book. It could be both a lifesaver and an exercise-restorer for you!

Okay, So Where Should You Begin?

You might feel overwhelmed thinking about starting aerobic, strength, and flexibility training all at once. For most people, though, the best way to begin is to *just get moving*! That's right: Just walk—outdoors, or indoors in a mall or elsewhere. Begin with one area and then add to it as you gain momentum.

Here's some good news too: Increasing your

physical activity is not as time-consuming as you might think. Studies show that in order to markedly improve your chances of avoiding diabetes you need to be active just 150 minutes (two and a half hours) over the course of a week. And interestingly, it doesn't appear to matter how you apportion that time. The same studies found that you achieve the same benefit whether you perform your 150 minutes all at once, work out for 50 minutes three times a week, or do 30 minutes of exercise five times a week. You get to pick! That's great news for the weekend warrior types, or those who simply can't fit in another thing during their workweek.

The type of activity you choose is also up to you. For example, a study published in *Diabetes Care* magazine found that the one-year incidence of type 2 diabetes for those considered to be at high risk for developing diabetes was reduced by *50 percent* in those who followed any one of the following exercise protocols:[3]

- 30 extra minutes per day of slow walking
- 20 extra minutes per day of brisk walking
- 10 extra minutes per day of jogging
- 5 extra minutes per day of jumping rope, playing basketball, or swimming

A quick calculation reveals that this marked health improvement didn't even require a full 150 minutes of activity. So you see, anything you do that raises your heart and breathing rate will be of benefit. Continuous yardwork, housecleaning, or speedy grocery shopping can count as minutes toward your exercise goal. Simply purpose to move more throughout your day. Take the stairs instead of the elevator, walk for 15 minutes during your lunch break, park your car farther away from the store's entrance—anything! Just make sure to move quickly enough to get a rise in your heart rate.

I find this very encouraging. A moderate commitment to get moving can ward off a lifetime of diabetes and its complications! Add to that the positive mental benefits—decreased stress, increased well-being/peace, and improved self-image—and you'll be batting a thousand—with blood sugar hopefully below 100.

Check In with Your Physician

It is always wise to seek clearance from your primary-care physician or cardiologist before beginning an exercise program. This is especially the case if you haven't had one before or know you have some medical issues that may warrant caution. The whole point of becoming more physically active is to improve your health, not compromise it.

A quick tip: I am more consistent and I exercise for a longer time when I invite a friend along (of course, this becomes a necessity if I'm going to play tennis). If you are social like me, think about who you might ask to join you. You'll find that you're more accountable and that the exercise is more enjoyable when someone else is involved. Another tip is to actually block out the time on your daily calendar. I know if I have something scheduled, I am more apt to follow through with it.

Take a few minutes right now to think about how you might best incorporate "moving on purpose" into your week. Jot it down in black-and-white—right here on this page if you need to. Sketch out a plan (days of the week and time of day) and begin (but see the sidebar above). Remember, you may need to modify your plan as you go. If you aren't sure you can do 150 minutes right off the bat, start slow and then build up.

The important thing is that you find something that works for you, By that I mean you enjoy the activity (at least somewhat), you have the time set aside for it, and you have "buddied up" (if need be) for better results. Happy trails to you—and don't be afraid to break a sweat. A little sweat lets you know you're hard at work! Tennis, anyone?

Chapter 10

Which Road Will You Choose?

Do you have any idea how much risk you feel comfortable taking? Likely it differs for each area of your life. You may feel quite comfortable speeding down the highway at 20 miles per hour above the limit, but you have all your money in safe investments. It may be a no-brainer to always monitor the whereabouts of your children, but it has been five years since your last complete checkup at your doctor's, and six months since you noticed that odd lump under your skin. Each of us has our own unique risk tolerance, and because people are generally fickle, many of us are quite inconsistent in the way we take chances in our lives.

The subtitle of this book indicates that one in three adults in the U.S. is afflicted with elevated blood sugar. Research confirms that your present risk of having diabetes or prediabetes is *33.3 percent,* or *one in three,* for adults over the age of 20. Next time you are seated in a theater or at church, look to the person on your left and the person on your right.

Statistically, one of the three of you is in trouble *today*.

Even though we've spoken about adults through most of this book, children in the U.S. are at even greater risk. It is estimated that 1 in 3 boys and 2 in 5 girls born in the year 2000 (today's ten-year-olds) will have *full-blown diabetes* in their lifetime.[1] (Even higher rates are projected for African-American and Hispanic populations.)

Let me ask you directly: How much risk, in terms of *your* physical well-being and longevity, are you willing to accept? If someone handed you a three-chambered pistol and told you they had placed a bullet in one chamber (1 in 3), how quick would you be to put that gun to your temple and pull the trigger? Chew on that awhile. There is no denying it—one in three adults in the U.S. will die (earlier than intended) suffering with the smorgasbord of diseases stemming from insulin resistance.

Below I'd like to share the stories of two different people as they journey through life.* Each has their own propensity for taking chances. Each makes certain choices based on that propensity. Their stories may help you sort out what your risk tolerance actually is.

---

* These characters have been fabricated from actual events experienced by my own patients and others.

Phyllis

People seemed to always form a circle around Phyllis. Her quick wit and bright smile would draw in the young and old, and even older. Around holidays, she was known as the hostess with the mostest. Her specialty dishes were tasty and packed with love—not to mention saturated fat! But oh, the flavor…

As she entered her forties, Phyllis began putting on weight—right in her middle, just like her mother had done years before. She seemed to steadily gain five more pounds a year, so by the time she turned 50, her bathroom scale told her she was a full 35 pounds heavier than on the day she was married. But Phyllis wasn't one to idle away her time thinking about herself much. Instead she was always busy working and meeting the needs of others—at her work, at church, and around home, where being a blessing to her husband, kids, and grandkids took priority.

As life sped by in all its fullness she awoke one day to find she had turned 62—ready for retirement—and was unfortunately a full 50 pounds heavier than she should be. Being a confident and determined woman, she set out to lose the weight that sat so uncomfortably around her middle. It was a battle, but like many goals she set for herself, she was successful. But only for a brief time. The weight she lost came back on faster than before. A year later her body looked exactly like it had before—like a big apple.

Phyllis began to notice other changes in her body—frequent trips to the bathroom to empty her bladder, tingling in her fingertips that would come and go, and blurriness in her eyesight. Finally concerned, she scheduled a long overdue appointment to see her physician. She sat speechless as he informed her that her blood pressure and glucose levels were both high—dangerously high. So she began her long-awaited retirement by popping pills, making more frequent trips to her doctors, and having more tests done in this decade of her life than in all the others put together!

On the morning of her sixty-fourth birthday Phyllis tested her blood glucose and it was 150—even though she was taking her medications every day. After another trip to the doctor and some more tests she was told she would have to begin insulin injections because the medication was not sufficiently controlling her blood sugar. Well, pills were one thing, but filling syringes of insulin and sticking herself with needles every day was not in line with Phyllis's fun-loving view of life. She was less than compliant with her doctor's orders—in fact, her compliancy problem even spread to her oral medications, and as a result her blood pressure was all over the map.

One day, while out shopping for a gift for her grandchild, Phyllis began to feel numbness in her left arm. Then she blacked out. The next time she was conscious she was in a hospital bed, surrounded by her family, unable to move the right side of her body. When she tried to speak to assure them she was all right, all her ears heard were mumbled incoherent sounds. Hot tears fell from her eyes as her family smiled sorrowfully back at her. Life was sadly altered for everyone in the room from that day forward.

Robert

Growing up in Texas, Robert ate, drank, and slept football. From the time he entered school as a young boy, afternoons and weekends were spent on the football field—whatever the weather. When he graduated high school, he went off to play ball at college on a partial scholarship. He had one disappointing season after another, and so his football "career" came to an end his senior year. However, he did accomplish one of his lifelong dreams—he was the first in his family to graduate from college.

Robert used his teaching degree to get himself a stable job at the local high school. For the next 20 years he made exercise a priority. Even if he couldn't play football any longer, he was determined to keep in shape. Three times a week he jogged five miles, and on alternate days he used his high school's weight machines to keep his muscles strong. Yet even with all this, by the time Robert turned 40, he found he'd collected a spare tire around his midsection. (Likely because he still ate the same amount of food he had back when playing college football.)

A week after his forty-second birthday he went to his doctor for his annual checkup. Much to Robert's surprise, when his doctor checked his glucose, he found his blood-sugar level was a little high and asked if Robert had eaten recently. Actually he was starving. He had missed lunch substituting for a colleague.

So Robert was sent to the lab the next morning to have a fasting glucose and a hemoglobin A1C test performed along with the usual blood work. A few days later his doctor's office called to schedule a follow-up. Robert knew something must be brewing even though he felt perfectly fine!

Thursday afternoon Robert heard the words that would change his life: *You have prediabetes.* He reacted. "What! How could I? I mean, I feel perfectly healthy." His doctor explained the problem of insulin resistance and pointed to his spare tire as a telltale sign of the metabolic problem. He then gave his patient two options: He could begin taking Metformin, a medication which would help to address the problem, or he could give Robert a chance to change his lifestyle first to see if he could make a change on his own.*

Robert was up to the challenge. Since he already had the exercise component down, the doctor suggested he read the books *Diabetes: Are You at Risk?* and *The South Beach Diet Supercharged.* Robert, still shell-shocked, wasted no time. He purchased both books on his drive home.

He devoured the books that very weekend, determined to find out how he could avoid medication, and even more important, how he could regain and maintain his health—which he had always valued. He realized he could have a positive effect on his blood sugar making by certain changes to his diet. Sadly, it required him to give up many of his "comfort foods"—bagels, French fries, potato chips, and Snickers bars. And he had to start limiting the amount of food he ate at each meal since, admittedly, he was no longer playing football two hours a day. His snacking habits had to change as well. Yet he continued to tell himself that he'd rather lose food options than years off his life.

Four months later Robert returned to his doctor's office following another round of blood tests. His fasting glucose was no longer elevated, and his A1C

---

* As mentioned earlier, the drug Metformin is effective in delaying or preventing the conversion of prediabetes to diabetes. However, it is not as effective as lifestyle intervention, which has been shown to reduce diabetes onset by 58 percent, while Metformin reduced its onset by only 31 percent.[2]

test findings had improved, though it was still not below 6.0. With these encouraging results, he continued his diet plan, which by now seemed quite normal to him. He was surprised that he no longer craved carbs like potato salad or cake. It was not hard now to pass on those once-tempting treats.

At his next doctor's visit, three months later, Robert's A1C test came back normal! And that was all the proof he needed to stay on track…for the rest of his life.

Did you see yourself, or parts of yourself, in either of those two accounts? As I write this chapter, a former patient of mine has just suffered a minor stroke. By his own admission, he had been playing roulette with his health for years. We had some very direct conversations about this while I was treating him for a shoulder injury. In fact, when I suggested he was likely prediabetic (he had two MBS markers and a "full belly"), he sat stunned. The next week he returned and thanked me sincerely for saying those hard-to-hear words. "No one ever used the term *prediabetic* with me. That got me scared—and motivated!"

He began on a new pathway to wellness that I had suggested during his last treatment session. He began losing weight, eating better, and exercising.

Yet his many years of neglecting his personal health, partnered with his strong family history of diabetes (both parents, and a sibling who had died from a diabetes-related stroke five years earlier) have obviously placed him at significant risk. I just pray this is the last wakeup call he'll need to stay on his new course toward better health. What about you—will you let this book be the only wakeup call you need?

When You Are "All Grown Up"

Researchers have polled today's teenagers about what they want to be when they grow up. Would it surprise you that the majority have been found to quickly respond "rich and famous"? (Not "a teacher" or "a doctor," as you might expect, right?) And while that might seem shallow, as adults, though we may not seek after fame per se, we do expend a great deal of our time and energy making money so we can accumulate things or experience pleasures that can be bought. We often live with little regard to the things that have no price tag—such as a healthy body.

While money does buy many things, it cannot buy all things. It cannot buy back your health once it has been lost. An older friend of mine, Marvin Jahn (who passed away recently), was known to say that if a problem could be fixed with money, then it wasn't a *true* problem after all.

If you think it through, Marvin was quite right.

In line with that premise, here's what an honest-to-goodness problem really is: losing your health, becoming dependent on medication and medical procedures for your survival, and ultimately succumbing to an insulin-resistance-related disease that can bring about your death many years earlier than your Maker intended!

The Blessing of Asher

Instead, my friend, I wish to give you one last thing before you lay this book down, something money cannot buy...the "blessing of Asher." These priceless words are found in an Old Testament book of the Bible, Deuteronomy. The blessing was spoken by the prophet Moses over one of the twelve tribes of Israel, descendents of a man by the name of Asher. In Deuteronomy 33:24-25, Moses offered the following prophetic proclamation: *"Most blessed of sons is Asher...your strength will equal your days."*

Now that is something money, talent, and opportunity simply cannot buy...a lifetime of physical strength. Given the choice, wouldn't we all want our strength to equal the number of days lived here on the earth? I know I do. As much as possible, I will work to avoid spending my latter years in an infirm body, a burden for those who must take care of me—all because I was too unmotivated or unconcerned to take better care of myself.

What's in a Name?

According to author and Bible teacher Beth Moore, throughout Scripture, there are two Hebrew words that are translated into English as "blessed." The first, *baruch,* is more accurately translated "to *be* blessed," whereas *asher* more precisely means "to *feel* blessed," or to feel happy. When your health is maintained, you will not only *be* blessed, but you will *feel* blessed as well!

It is my sincere hope that you too will love yourself, your family, and your friends enough to take care of yourself...and to stay alive for all your intended days in an effort to bless the next generation. My friend, may this book motivate and encourage you to do what you can. Take hold of the blessing of Asher. May you live long and be strong until your final day.

Stay true to yourself
and to your calling.
—Lisa

Resources

National Diabetes Information Clearinghouse (NDIC)
1 Information Way
Bethesda, MD 20892-3560
Phone: 1-800-860-8747 (TTY: 1-866-569-1162)
www.diabetes.niddk.nih.gov

American Diabetes Association (ADA)
www.diabetes.org

American Association of Clinical Endocrinologists (AACE)
Downloadable Diabetes Passport to take to your doctor visits:
www.aace.com/documents/pdf/DiabetesPassport.pdf

The South Beach Diet Supercharged, Arthur Agatston, M.D.

Home Blood-Test Sources (as of April 2010)

- The ADA CheckUp America American Diabetes Association Cholesterol Panel, available at www.drugstore.com.
- Bayer's A1CNow SELFCHECK System, available at CVS, Walmart, and Walgreen pharmacies.

Notes

Headed for Trouble?

1. Centers for Disease Control and Prevention (CDC), "Frequently Asked Questions: Preventing Diabetes," www.cdc.gov/diabetes/faq/prediabetes.htm, accessed 2009 March 19; W.H. Herman, T.J. Hoerger, M. Brandle, et al. "The Cost-Effectiveness of Lifestyle Modification or Metformin in Preventing Type 2 Diabetes in Adults with Impaired Glucose Tolerance," *Annals of Internal Medicine,* 2005; 142:323-332.

Chapter 1—Sweet but Deadly

1. E-medicine from WebMD, Medscape, "Diabetes Mellitus, Type 2—Review," April 7, 2009, http://emedicine.medscape.com/article/766143-overview.
2. American Diabetes Association, "Direct and Indirect Costs of Diabetes in the United States," www.diabetes.org/diabetes-statistics/cost-of-diabetes-in-us.jsp, accessed 2009 April 15.
3. Yale University School of Medicine, *Diabetes 2009,* April 1, 2009 (vol. 19, p.1), as quoted in newsletter from the 58th Annual Scientific Sessions of the American College of Cardiology, Orlando, FL.
4. E-medicine from WebMD.
5. National Diabetes Information Clearinghouse (NDIC), "National Diabetes Statistics 2007," http://diabetes.niddk.nih.gov/dm/pubs/statistics/#allages, accessed 2009 April 7.
6. National Diabetes Information Clearinghouse.
7. E-medicine from WebMD.
8. Zachary T. Bloomgarden, "Insulin resistance syndrome and nonalcoholic fatty liver disease," *Diabetes Care,* 2005 (28:1518-1523).

Chapter 2—Do You Fit the Profile?

1. *New York Times,* "Health Guide, Type 2 Diabetes," April 16, 2009, http://health.nytimes.com/health/guides/disease/type-2-diabetes/risk-factors.html.

2. E-medicine from WebMD, Medscape, "Diabetes Mellitus, Type 2—Review," April 7, 2009, http://emedicine.medscape.com/article/766143-overview.

3. National Diabetes Information Clearinghouse (NDIC), "National Diabetes Statistics 2007," http://diabetes.niddk.nih.gov/dm/pubs/statistics/#race, accessed 2009 April 16.

4. *New York Times,* "Health Guide."

5. National Diabetes Information Clearinghouse (NDIC), "National Diabetes Statistics 2007," http://diabetes.niddk.nih.gov/dm/pubs/statistics/ #allages, accessed 2009 April 7.

Chapter 3—What Goes Up Must Come Down

1. Scott Isaacs and Frederic J. Vagnini, *Overcoming Metabolic Syndrome* (Omaha, NE: Addicus Books, Inc., 2006), p. 4.

2. Endocrineweb, "Endocrine Tumors of the Pancreas: A Patient Information Guide to Insulin, Glucagon, Somatostatin and Gastrin," May 21, 2009, www.endocrineweb.com/insulin.html.

3. James Norman, "Normal Regulation of Blood Glucose: The Important Roles of Insulin and Glucagon," May 22, 2009, www.endocrineweb.com/insulin.html.

Chapter 4—The Road to Diabetes

1. Lisa Morrone, *Overcoming Overeating* (Eugene, OR: Harvest House Publishers, 2009).

Chapter 5—Is Diabetes in Your Future?

1. W.H. Herman, T.J. Hoerger, M. Brandle, et al. "The Cost-Effectiveness of Lifestyle Modification or Metformin in Preventing Type 2 Diabetes in Adults with Impaired Glucose Tolerance," *Annals of Internal Medicine,* 2005; 142:323-332.

2. Scott Isaacs and Frederic J. Vagnini, *Overcoming Metabolic Syndrome* (Omaha, NE: Addicus Books, Inc., 2006), p. 12.

3. Gabriel Hilkovitz, *Preventing Type 2 Diabetes* (Scottsdale, AZ: Bel Vista Publishers, LLC, 2008), p. 31.

4. Dungan et al., *Diabetes Care,* 2006; 29(6):1214-1219.

Chapter 6—Am I at Risk?

1. Johns Hopkins Bloomberg School of Public Health, "Waist Size Linked to Diabetes Risk in Adult Men," *ScienceDaily,* March 28, 2005, www.sciencedaily.com/releases/2005/03/050325150149.htm, accessed September 16, 2009.

2. University of California, Los Angeles, "Waist-hip Ratio Better than BMI for Gauging Obesity in Elderly, Study Finds." *ScienceDaily,* September 2, 2009, www.sciencedaily.com/releases/2009/09/090901150951.htm, accessed September 16, 2009.

Chapter 7—Marshmallows for Dinner

1. Scott Isaacs and Frederic J. Vagnini, *Overcoming Metabolic Syndrome* (Omaha, NE: Addicus Books, Inc., 2006), pp. 65, 68.

2. Isaacs and Vagnini, p. 70.

3. Cheryle Hart and Mary Kay Grossman, *The Insulin-Resistant Diet* (New York: McGraw-Hill, 2008), pp. 31-34.

4. Hart and Grossman, pp. 39-44.

5. Jack Challem, *Stop Prediabetes Now* (Hoboken, NJ: John Wiley & Sons, Inc., 2007), p. 91.

6. Challem, p. 88.

7. Arthur Agatston, *The South Beach Diet Supercharged* (New York: Rodale, Inc., 2008), pp. 174-182.

Chapter 8—More Than Enough

1. Michèle Guerre-Millo, "Adipose tissue hormones," *The Journal of Endocrinology Investigation,* 2002; 25:855-861.

2. Lisa Morrone, *Overcoming Overeating* (Eugene, OR: Harvest House Publishers, 2009), pp. 161-163.

3. B. Wansink, J.E. Painter, and J. North, "Bottomless Bowls: Why Visual Cues of Portion Size May Influence Intake," *Obesity Research,* 2005; 13(1):93-100.

4. B. Wansink, K. Van Ittersum, J.E. Painter, "Ice Cream Illusions:

Bowls, Spoons, and Self-Served Portion Sizes," *American Journal of Preventive Medicine,* 2006; 31(3):240-243.

Chapter 9–"Ex"-Rated

1. W.H. Herman, T.J. Hoerger, M. Brandle, et al. "The Cost-Effectiveness of Lifestyle Modification or Metformin in Preventing Type 2 Diabetes in Adults with Impaired Glucose Tolerance," *Annals of Internal Medicine,* 2005; 142:323-332; F. DeVegt, J.M. Dekker, A. Jager, et al., "Relations of impaired fasting and post-load glucose with incident type 2 diabetes in a Dutch population: The Hoorn Study," *Journal of American Medicine,* 2001; 285:2109-2113.

2. J.O. Holloszy, "Exercise-induced increase in muscle insulin sensitivity," *The Journal of Applied Physiology,* July 2005; 99(1):338-43.

3. K. Yamaoka and T. Tango, "Efficacy of lifestyle education to prevent type 2 diabetes: A meta-analysis of randomized controlled trials," *Diabetes Care,* 2005; 28:2780-2786.

Chapter 10–Which Road Will You Choose?

1. Centers for Disease Control and Prevention (CDC), "Frequently Asked Questions: Preventing Diabetes," www.cdc.gov/diabetes/faq/prediabetes.htm, accessed April 7, 2009.

2. W.C. Knowler, E. Barrett-Conner, S.E. Fowler, et al., "The Diabetes Prevention Program Research Group: Reduction in the incidence of type 2 diabetes with lifestyle intervention or Metformin," *New England Journal of Medicine,* 2002; 344:393-403.

More Life-Changing Help from Lisa Morrone and Harvest House Publishers

OVERCOMING BACK AND NECK PAIN
A Proven Program for Recovery and Prevention

From 20 years of teaching and practicing physical therapy, Lisa Morrone gives you a way to say *no* to the treadmill of prescriptions, endless treatments, and a limited lifestyle. This straightforward, clinically proven approach shows you how to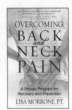

- strengthen and stretch key muscles and shift to healthy movement patterns
- recover from pain caused by compressed or degenerated discs
- address "inside issues" that affect healing—nutrition, rest, and emotional/spiritual struggles

OVERCOMING HEADACHES AND MIGRAINES
Clinically Proven Cure for Chronic Pain

Physical therapist Lisa Morrone offers a thorough, broad-based perspective on head pain. She helps you discover how to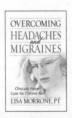

- uncover the *source* of your head pain and avoid unnecessary medication
- eliminate pain originating from neck problems or muscle tension
- ward off migraines and cluster headaches by pinpointing and avoiding your "triggers"
- find a qualified hands-on practitioner

OVERCOMING OVEREATING
It's Not What You Eat, It's What's Eating You!

Health author Lisa Morrone bypasses diet plans and zeros in on *heart* plans—because food isn't typically the real problem. Here are tools to assess *yourself* (not just your food intake), followed by tested methods for breaking through the food trap from the inside out. You'll find ways to

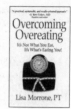

- identify and address the underlying causes of your overeating
- avoid using food as a time-filler, mood elevator, or painkiller
- find freedom to achieve steady, solid results from any reputable weight-loss method
- *finally* keep the weight off, feel better about yourself, and improve your overall health

TAKING CHARGE OF YOUR OWN HEALTH
Navigating Your Way Through Diagnosis • Treatment • Insurance

LISA HALL, WITH RONALD M. WYATT, MD, MHA

When you face a health-care need today, you have to be prepared for

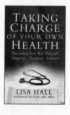

- less personal attention
- more complications with insurance and government programs
- a *40 percent national misdiagnosis rate,* per recent surveys

Author Lisa Hall can help. Her years-long search for diagnosis has given her top-to-bottom experience with the health-care system. Aided by the expertise of internal-medicine doctor

Ronald Wyatt, Lisa provides a wide variety of practical guidance on how to

- find the right kind of doctor, check qualifications, and increase the benefits of office visits
- navigate medical insurance, Medicare, workers' compensation, and Social Security disability
- avoid being a victim of hospital mistakes
- organize your medical records in a way that helps practitioners help *you*

When you take charge of your own health, you'll be ready to proactively take advantage of the help that's out there.

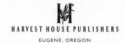